OUR HANDS
ARE TIED

Legal Tensions and
Medical Ethics

Marshall B. Kapp

AUBURN HOUSE
Westport, Connecticut
London

Library of Congress Cataloging-in-Publication Data

Kapp, Marshall B.
  Our hands are tied : legal tensions and medical ethics / Marshall
B. Kapp.
    p.   cm.
  Includes bibliographical references and index.
  ISBN 0-86569-276-9 (alk. paper)
  1. Physicians—Malpractice—United States. 2. Adversary system
(Law)—United States. 3. Medical ethics—United States. I. Title.
KF2905.3.K37   1998
344.73′04121—DC21   97-38581

British Library Cataloguing in Publication Data is available.

Library of Congress Catalog Card Number: 97-38581
ISBN: 0-86569-276-9

First published in 1998

Auburn House, 88 Post Road West, Westport, CT 06881
An imprint of Greenwood Publishing Group, Inc.

Printed in the United States of America

The paper used in this book complies with the
Permanent Paper Standard issued by the National
Information Standards Organization (Z39.48-1984).

10 9 8 7 6 5 4 3 2 1

To the Memory of H. R. K. and B. B. K.
"You shouldn't make excuses."

Contents

Preface   ix

Acknowledgments   xv

1. Losing at the Lottery: Physician Perceptions
   of the Legal Environment   1

2. The Lawyer Made Me Do It: From Legal Perception
   to Medical Practice   27

3. Risk Managers and Legal Counsel: Ethical Enablers
   or Paid Paranoids?   53

4. Doing Everything: Treating Legal Fears near the End of Life   65

5. Who Is Responsible for This? Everyday Patient Intrusions
   to Protect the Provider   97

6. "A Dispirited Lot": Malpractice and What Else?   123

7. Reconciling Risk Management and Medical Ethics:
   Opportunities and Obstacles   141

Index   171

Preface

"The practice patterns of individual clinicians are fundamental determinants of the quality, ethical standards, and cost-effectiveness of health services" (Logan & Scott, 1996, p. 595). Physicians' practice patterns are influenced by a wide variety of factors, both conscious and subconscious. For at least the last century and a half, physicians have insisted that one of those factors—mainly negative in effect—is the pervasive anxiety and apprehension physicians experience about potential malpractice litigation and legal liability connected to the care that they provide to their patients (Mohr, 1993, pp. 109–121; Wachsman, 1993, p. 161).

Physicians as well as other health care professionals in the United States are constantly complaining about lawyers and the persistent possibility of being held legally liable for decisions made and actions taken in the course of caring for patients. The vast majority of practicing physicians have long told anyone who would listen that apprehension about potential litigation and liability influences medical professionals to practice "defensively," and therefore wastefully in an economic sense.

Although they are nothing new, these complaints lately have intensified in bitterness and broadened in scope. The primary claim used to focus on the financial waste entailed in practicing defensive medicine.

More recently, though, one is likely to hear the lament that binding legal dictates (that is, the need for physicians as well as other health care providers to specially tailor their conduct to avoid litigation and liability) often act in opposition not only to cost containment precepts but to good clinical judgment and accepted principles of medical ethics also.

THE ETHICAL LOBOTOMIZING OF THE HEALTH PROFESSIONS

As an attorney working in a medical education setting, I am exposed to these laments frequently. As I contemplate their significance, I have grown increasingly disturbed about the medical paradigm of "ethical lobotomy" in which too many physicians appear influenced in their daily decisions and actions far less by a thoughtful consideration of ethical principles and consequences than by calculations for avoiding regulatory and judicial sanctions. This ethical lobotomy is an essential part of the "our hands are tied" syndrome from which a growing segment of the medical profession seems to suffer. The result can be a "deprofessionalization" of medicine in which medical judgment is willingly forfeited in return for protection against public accountability (Annas, 1996).

The relationship between law and ethics as applied to medical practice varies depending on the particular circumstances involved. In specific cases, law and ethics may be synonymous, distinct, at odds, complementary, or overlapping. An analysis of the law-ethics relationship is complicated markedly by the often enormous chasms between three distinct approaches to the law, namely: (a) the law "in books" (how law professors and appellate judges describe the law); (b) the law "in the mind" (how physicians imagine, fear, and frequently caricature the law); and (c) the law "in action" (the way in which clinicians actually practice because of or in spite of their perceptions about the law) (Schuck, 1994, p. 903).

When the law in the physician's mind conflicts or is inconsistent with her concept of what is ethical under the circumstances, almost always the legal concerns crowd out the ethical ones when the physician's calculations are translated into action (De Ville, 1994a). Physicians believe (most of the time erroneously) that the law provides definitive guidance in concrete situations, unlike "soft" and "fuzzy" ethics. Further, physicians believe that they may be forced to endure bad, tangible, concrete consequences if second-guessed legally but not if criticized on ethical grounds.

Unfortunately, this displacement of ethics by perceived risk management needs occurs regularly in actual practice, despite the poor capacity of legislatures and courts to guide participants about, let alone satisfactorily resolve, ethical dilemmas. As one commentator has noted, "By their nature, courts [and legislators often, too] deal with medical relationships gone wrong. This raw material for medicolegal doctrine engenders a frame of reference and precedents that frequently misapprehend the nature of the medical relationship" (De Ville, 1994a, p. 479). The President's Commission for the Study of Ethical Problems in Medicine and Biomedical and Behavioral Research concluded that "its vision of the patient-professional relationship" cannot be achieved "primarily through reliance on the law" (President's Commission, 1982, p. 152).

Bioethics pioneer Daniel Callahan has suggested that the greatest obstacle to outright and serious public moral debate in this country is "the hovering presence of the law." He warns, "The danger in our country of opening moral discussions about private matters is that some one or other is likely to have the idea that 'there ought to be a law.'" Callahan attacks "legalism," which he defines "as the translation of moral problems into legal problems; the inhibition of moral debate for fear that it will be so translated; and the elevation of the moral judgments of courts as the moral standards of the land" (Callahan, 1996, p. 34).

In commenting on the dynamics between law and ethics in the crucible of medical care, one observer has perceptively concluded that ultimately "one's choice of protective measures is itself a vexing ethical problem" (De Ville, 1994b, p. 193). It is the problem that forms the core of this book.

WHY AND HOW?

Provoked by the sort of claims just described, and with the financial support of the Greenwall Foundation, I decided to investigate in depth the defensive medicine phenomenon, concentrating particularly on the influence that apprehension about litigation and legal liability exerts on ethical medical practice today. I wanted to pay special attention to the real and perceived tensions between risk management and defensive medicine, on one hand, and good (i.e., ethical) patient care, on the other. The aim of this book is a critical examination of the "our hands are tied" syndrome, not for the purpose of defending lawyers or the current legal system in the United States, but rather to place in some realistic perspective the impact—actual and ideal—of legal principles on modern medical decision making and treatment.

Among the specific questions I set out to explore through literature review, personal interviews of physicians and observers of the medical profession, and primarily reflection on lessons learned during my more than decade and a half working and teaching in medical environments, were the following:

What is the etiology of the anxiety about litigation and liability that appears to pervade American medical practice in the 1990s? Put differently, where do modern physicians get their notions about what the law forbids, requires, and punishes?

How much physician apprehension in this sphere is well-founded and how much emanates from misunderstanding or mythology? Is the apprehension free-floating or predicated on specific, real experiences? What particular beliefs do physicians hold about the legal environment, versus a generalized feeling of malaise?

How do physician perceptions about legal requirements, prohibitions, and potential adversities manifest themselves in patient care situations? Do physicians perceive these behavioral manifestations as positive or as interfering with their ability to practice ethically?

If a tension exists between defensive medicine and ethical medical practice, what can be done to mitigate or resolve that tension? What changes would encourage medical practice that more closely incorporates the ethical values that are now sometimes jeopardized by that tension?

This volume represents the fruits of my investigation. In Chapter 1, physician attitudes toward the law, and especially regarding the current system for handling medical malpractice lawsuits, are analyzed. This includes discussion of the origins of physicians' legal fears, the expectations of certainty and infallibility that physicians impose upon themselves, and what physicians believe the public wants of them and the health care enterprise. Chapter 2 outlines both salutary and deleterious effects of defensive medicine on the ethical quality of care provided to patients, primarily in the context of medical decisions about the use of various diagnostic and therapeutic interventions. The concept of "defensive medicine as pretext for something else" is raised at this juncture.

Chapter 3 comments on physician perceptions about the roles and influence on clinical practice of health care risk managers and legal counsel. The relationship between risk management and institutional ethics committees and ethics consultants is also broached here.

Chapter 4 looks specifically at the ways that provider apprehension about civil, criminal, and regulatory liability often encourages tragic overly aggressive, even cruel, interventions to be inflicted on seriously ill and dying patients. Chapter 5 contains a discussion of paternalistic defensive medicine as it limits patient prerogatives in such areas as assisted living, guardianship, and involuntary commitment. Chapter 6 assesses the likely impact of managed care and other emerging changes in the American health care financing and delivery system on the defensive medicine / medical ethics interface.

The book concludes with a look at possible solutions to the problem of defensive medicine interfering with ethical medical practice. Proposals for initiatives in public policy (e.g., tort reform), professional education, and organizational activity (e.g., the development and dissemination of clinical practice parameters) are set forth for consideration.

This volume articulates my own conjectures and conclusions, supported where possible by references to the professional and popular literature. Statements denoted by quotation marks represent, unless otherwise noted, direct quotes from individuals with whom I have spoken about the topics discussed herein.

Careful study and dissection of the defensive medicine phenomenon in the United States have been woefully inadequate to date. In the course of assembling this project, I interviewed the coauthor of one of the few nationally recognized legitimate analyses in this field. In reply to my query about how he had become an expert on defensive medicine, he joked, "It was easy. I wrote an article on the topic twenty years ago, and every night I reread it." Defensive medicine and its impact on medical ethics is no joke, however; it is a serious matter compelling serious attention.

Nobel Prize winner Aleksandr Solzhenitsyn lectured the 1978 Harvard graduating class. He said that although a society without an objective legal scale is terrible, "a society with no other scale but the legal one is not quite worthy of man either":

> A society that is based on the letter of the law and never reaches any higher is taking very small advantages of the high level of human possibilities. The letter of the law is too cold and formal to have a beneficial influence on society. Whenever the tissue of life is woven of legalistic relations, there is an atmosphere of mediocrity, paralysing man's noblest impulse. (Solzhenitsyn, 1978, p. 22)

In the context of medical care, it is the noblest impulse of human nature to treat the patient and family with dignity, respect, and loving kindness. Many physicians believe that "[t]he law, however, has no philosophical construct for kindness and is, therefore, unable to provide for the logical incorporation of kindness into its formulations and promulgations" (Frengley, 1996, p. 1126). Although that sentiment overstates the case a bit, its author is correct in exhorting, "It behooves physicians to challenge our legal colleagues and to insist that kindness be one of the values that guide the practice of medicine" (Frengley, 1996, p. 1126).

Effective risk management and legal prophylaxis need not necessarily conflict with medicine's noble impulse. This book is my modest attempt to contribute to a better understanding of the impact of defensive medicine on ethical practice and to the identification of effective strategies for accomplishing the valid goals of legal regulation of health care delivery without impairing the ability to respect fundamental ethical values.

I have suggested in some earlier writings that the law, as the current best expression of society's values and authority regarding specific issues, may not be ignored, but neither should it automatically dictate disregard of other important sources of those values. It is the constellation of values from a broad range of perspectives, law included but by no means alone, that ought to guide those who have undertaken the awesome clinical and ethical obligations of patient well-being. It is the goal of this book to make physicians feel safer to recognize and respect that rich constellation of values, and thereby to practice medicine more ethically. It is my hope that "[f]or a change, law may be the handmaiden of ethics and ethics served by the law rather than vice versa" (Abrams & Veenhuis, 1986, p. 9).

REFERENCES

Abrams, R. A., & Veenhuis, P. (1986). Ethical questions raised by a proposed randomized, double-blind study involving placebo, standard drug therapy, and experimental antipsychotic drug therapy for patients with schizophrenia. *Clinical Research, 34,* 6–9.

Annas, G. J. (1996). Facilitating choice: Judging the physician's role in abortion and suicide. *Quinnipiac Health Law Journal, 1,* 93–112.

Callahan, D. (1996, November–December). Escaping from legalism: Is it possible? *Hastings Center Report, 26,* 34–35.

De Ville, K. (1994a). "What does the law say?" Law, ethics and medical decision making. *Western Journal of Medicine, 160,* 478–480.

De Ville, K. (1994b). Response to letter. *Western Journal of Medicine, 161,* 192–193.

Frengley, J. D. (1996). The use of physical restraints and the absence of kindness. *Journal of the American Geriatrics Society, 44,* 1125–1127.

Logan, R. L., & Scott, P. J. (1996). Uncertainty in clinical practice: Implications for quality and costs of health care. *Lancet, 347,* 595–598.

Mohr, J. C. (1993). *Doctors and the law: Medical jurisprudence in nineteenth-century America.* New York: Oxford University Press.

President's Commission for the Study of Ethical Problems in Medicine and Biomedical and Behavioral Research (1982). *Making health care decisions,* vol. 1. Washington, DC: U.S. Government Printing Office.

Schuck, P. H. (1994). Rethinking informed consent. *Yale Law Journal, 103,* 899–959.

Solzhenitsyn, A. (1978). The exhausted West. *Harvard Magazine, 82*(6), 22.

Wachsman, H. F. (1993). *Lethal medicine: The epidemic of medical malpractice in America.* New York: Henry Holt and Company.

Acknowledgments

My sincere appreciation is extended to the Greenwall Foundation for its financial support of this project. Many of the ideas that animated this project originated during a Robert Wood Johnson Foundation Fellowship in Health Care Finance that I enjoyed in 1987–88, particularly the facet in which I had the opportunity to learn more about medical malpractice public policy as a "fly on the wall" in the Office of the Undersecretary of the U.S. Department of Health and Human Services; my research grant from the Greenwall Foundation almost a decade later allowed me to explore these ideas in an organized fashion. For the many busy physicians, attorneys, ethicists, and others who provided me with data—through personal interviews, correspondence, and feedback during a number of formal presentations I had the opportunity to make during the course of this project—I extend my thanks for your time and insights; considerations of confidentiality prevent me from identifying you individually here, but you know who you are. As usual, the staff of the Fordham Health Sciences Library at Wright State University was extremely helpful in locating materials and in holding my hand while I entered the age of computerized databases kicking and screaming. Christina DeWitt provided her usual reliable secretarial support.

Losing at the Lottery: Physician Perceptions of the Legal Environment

INTRODUCTION—PHYSICIAN ATTITUDES TOWARD LEGAL RISK

Legal tensions profoundly affect physicians' ethical conduct in every-day medical practice. To comprehend this dynamic, one must begin with some understanding of physician attitudes toward their own legal risks. These attitudes are best summed up as a professional ethos of zero legal risk tolerance, reinforced continually by an almost "Pavlovian hostility toward [the] law" (Williams & Winslade, 1995, p. 783). Physicians' view of the universe as a scary and dangerous legal place for them and their patients has become such a commonplace and automatic assumption (Ferguson, 1993; Wolter, 1993) that I half expect tomorrow's newspapers to trumpet the discovery of an "anti-lawyer" gene that predisposes carriers to pursue medical careers.

Repeatedly and vigorously, physicians indicate that their primary anxiety about legal system entanglement is fear of the traumatic experience of being civilly sued for malpractice,[1] an event which they interpret as a deeply personal and intimate, yet simultaneously an embarrassingly public affront against their very integrity and worth as professionals and as people. In terms of the psychological and financial trauma that they fear, few physicians seem to distinguish (in other than purely intellectual terms, perhaps) between the experience of being sued, on one hand, and the ability to defend successfully against a malpractice lawsuit, on the other. Put differently, most physicians feel that they have already "lost" the sense of self-confidence and peer respect that they value most highly upon the mere filing of a malpractice action against them, regardless of the ultimate legal and financial outcome of that claim (McQuade, 1991). Living through the legal process itself is more intimidating than the specific financial result (which, even at the worst, ordinarily is taken care of by sufficient liability insurance).

This attitude about the very act of being named a defendant in a malpractice case makes most physicians highly risk-averse in terms of their own perceived legal exposure. This acute risk-aversion, in turn, potentially confers a substantial degree of power on those—such as risk managers (see Chapter 3)—who physicians believe can affect their susceptibility to being sued for professional wrongdoing.

Virtually every practicing physician wants to behave toward patients in good faith—that is, competently and ethically. A clinician's good faith behavior may be called into question by: external entities, most significantly one's own patients and the legal system; one's professional peers; and, ultimately, the physician himself or herself (Bosk, 1979, pp. 170–171).

In this chapter, I endeavor to lay the analytical groundwork for the ethical evaluation of specific manifestations of defensive medicine that follows in subsequent chapters. I first speculate about physician conceptions of what the public wants and expects from modern American medicine, with special emphasis on what physicians surmise they need to do in order to please their individual patients and—sometimes even more importantly in terms of risk management—their families. This leads naturally to an exploration of physician attitudes and understandings regarding the legal system as the other (along with individual patients) most important external entity functioning in the role of constant overseer and potential critic. Next, I offer informed hypotheses about the etiology of physicians' law-related anxieties. I ask specifically where physicians manage to come up with their ideas—so often factually erroneous—regarding the particular medical conduct required, permitted, or forbidden by that mysterious and engulfing black hole, "the law." Finally, I prepare the way for ensuing sections by examining the major expectations and standards that physicians impose upon themselves and their colleagues, including a brief notice of how the concepts of medical error and uncertainty fundamentally affect medical professionals' careers and lives.

WHAT DO THEY WANT OF ME?

Patients and Their Families

Overwhelmingly, physicians believe that their patients want their professional caregivers to "do things" to them and, moreover, that the public has been conditioned to believe that more—and more expensive—medical intervention is virtually always preferable to less-intrusive and cheaper strategies (Wright, 1995). Modern patients, according to this portrait of the medical environment, almost insatiably demand and expect a constant barrage of tests, procedures, and prescriptions. The medical profession, as well as its social critics (Annas, 1996, p. 105), decry the fact that today's physicians too often have been reduced in moral stature from the role of professional exercising appropriate judgment and discretion to that of "provider" responding to "consumer demands" personified by patients "showing up for appointments with articles in their fists." Most physicians complain about feeling pressured, both by the competitive marketplace with its premium on hustling for patients and by the fear of potential malpractice suits brought by disgruntled individuals, to accede too often to scientifically unreasonable patient (or family) requests to render particular purported diagnostic or therapeutic treatments of questionable, if any, likely benefit to the patient.

Assuming that physicians are correct on this matter (which is by no means a foregone conclusion [Britten, 1995]), these complaints still must be evaluated carefully in light of how closely and compatibly patient expectations and desires for maximum medical intervention comport with the technological, data-glorification imperative into which medical practitioners become thoroughly socialized and the economic incentives that, until the recent ascension of managed care (see Chapter 6), influenced physicians to overtreat patients as a way to maximize payments to providers. Skepticism should be heightened by a realization that modern public images of medicine and its unlimited capabilities emanate not only from fantasies projected by the entertainment industry and unsophisticated, ill-informed snippets in the popular press and other media. These images emanate as well from the successful "selling job" that the medical profession itself has accomplished on the public.

Most physicians acknowledge, albeit often begrudgingly, their own individual and collective roles in creating the success—that is, in convincing the public of medicine's magic—of which they are now partially victims. A few are still in deep denial, however. After attending a professional conference on the medical malpractice problem in another city not long ago, I rode in a van to the airport with several physicians I had just met. I called to their attention the irony of a billboard we passed that advertised the "laser perfect" results patients could expect if they indulged in cosmetic services from a particular local plastic surgeon. One of my medical vanmates failed to grasp the irony, proclaiming that "since everyone knows that health care advertising is filled with lies anyway, no reasonable person would believe that billboard." The upshot of his argument was that health providers ought to be permitted to advertise the quality of their services (i.e., to tell lies to people who know they are being lied to) but should not be held accountable for the substance of those lies. Although not exactly the most ringing endorsement of the present health care industry in the United States by one of its participants, this physician's cynical special pleading was, unfortunately, hardly an example of an isolated mind-set.

With this larger historical and social context before us, then, we cannot avoid asking to what extent physician lamentations about unreasonable patient expectations function primarily as a pretext (conscious or not) used by physicians to rationalize conduct (i.e., excessive medical intervention) that really has other, less publicly acceptable, motives at its core (Sox & Nease, 1993). This "legal anxiety as pretext" theme is one that I will refer to repeatedly throughout this volume.

However we resolve that part of the puzzle, every physician certainly endures a certain proportion of unpleasant patients and families. Most physicians, of course, want to maintain positive fiduciary or trust relationships with their patients and patients' family members as a central element of the general satisfaction inspiring a medical career in the first place. As noted previously, though, there also are two externally induced reasons that physicians now feel more of a need to attend to the quality of these relationships: namely, (a) the need to compete for insured "customers" in the brave new world of managed care, and (b) the fear that unhappy partners (including in many situations family members) in the physician-patient relationship may play out their frustrations in the context of malpractice litigation. These forces for short-term appeasement of patients and families who make unreasonable demands for medical interventions, even when the more honest and beneficent physician reaction would be to devote the time and effort needed to educate and convince them otherwise, frequently are reinforced by administrative officials when the scenario unfolds (as it usually does) within an institutional or organizational setting.

Though a small percentage of both patients and physicians probably permit thoughts—conscious or unconscious—about possible litigation to infuse every aspect of each medical encounter, for the majority such a constant state of extreme vigilance would be exhausting to the point of rendering them dysfunctional. Although some physicians "see a lawsuit every time a patient walks through the door," for most the threat of litigation is omnipresent but only at the level of "background noise." One neurosurgeon advises his colleagues to treat this threat "as they would a chronic skin disease, seldom fatal but always nettlesome, never sure where the next eruption will appear, and for which one forgoes the hope of cure and seeks, at most, a means to cope" (Davey, 1990, p. 210).

But background noise in many instances can be quite loud and even deafening when the physician (as every physician periodically does) "smells" a souring relationship with a patient or family. Physicians are uniformly convinced that any of their patients would, under the "right" circumstances, adopt an "entitlement mentality" and turn on them legally. Most physicians are under the impression that to the extent that patients ever think about these matters proactively, their patients subscribe to an unseen but lingering notion that the threat of litigation serves the inevitably positive purpose of assuring quality care by "keeping physicians on their toes."

More specifically, patients on the whole are seen as far less worried about the potential excesses and risks of defensive medicine than about the possibility of being cheated out of adequate attention because of the physician's financial incentives to skimp under managed care. One hears few stories of patients and families telling the physician, "Please be conservative in your diagnostic and treatment plan, and we won't sue you if you miss an opportunity that turns out later to be significant." The opposite scenario—"Miss something and we'll sue you"—is much easier to envision. This patient attitude is natural, given the extent to which organized medicine and individual physicians have both publicly and privately savaged the idea and the implementation of marketplace-driven health care and lobbied for legislative protections from it (see Chapter 6), at a level just as vicious as the medical community had previously risen to in bashing the possibility of government-driven health care and its excessive legislative entanglements.

Lawyers and "Their" System

In light of the previous discussion, physicians' concerns about unreasonable and unsatisfied (and often inherently unsatisfiable) expectations among patients and their families spills directly into concerns about lawyers and the legal system. There is a bit of variation among different medical specialties and practice settings in terms of the intensity of legal apprehension; oncologists, for instance, ordinarily are somewhat less on edge about liability risks than many of their counterparts (McCrary, Swanson, Perkins, & Winslade, 1992, p. 369) because most cancer patients come to them "with hopes but not high expectations." Despite this variation, physicians' general attitudes toward lawyers and the medical malpractice part of the legal system well-nigh approach a monolithic character—"We are swimming in a pool of sharks."

Those attitudes coalesce around the bedrock belief that the current (and quite long-standing) civil tort system for adjudicating claims of medical malpractice is unpredictable and, therefore, at its heart unfair. This almost universally shared opinion of unfairness probably is the worst indictment that could be brought against the existing legal system; people can manage to live with almost any substantive legal result as long as they feel they have been treated equitably by the process through which the decision was reached (Tyler, 1990, pp. 146–148). Lack of confidence in the system's fairness, however, sows the seeds of anarchy.

Anarchy or chaos (Konner, 1993, p. xx) is precisely the image that most American physicians would use to describe the prevailing tort system. Medical practitioners readily indicate to whoever will listen that they "want to believe the worst about the law," and they do. Physicians overwhelmingly see malpractice litigation as a haphazard form of "random event," "lottery" (Berczeller, 1994, p. 210), "roulette game," or "bolt of lightning" over which neither the defendant nor any other reasonable party has any control. They describe the legal environment as "'the malpractice equivalent of Beirut'—an image of relentless and often pointless crossfire" (Konner, 1993, pp. 18–19) and a state of "global unrest" that "turns doctors into near-paranoids" (Howard, 1996). The system is envisioned as "without restraint or accountability."

Moreover, physicians almost uniformly reject any justification of the current legal system that attempts to link litigation to quality assurance, believing instead that the quality of medical care actually provided is, for all intents and purposes, irrelevant in predicting whether a malpractice suit will be brought by a dissatisfied patient or family and how such a suit will ultimately be resolved (Brennan, Sox, & Burstin, 1996; Brennan & Berwick, 1996, pp. 190–191; Localio, Lawthers, Brennan, Laird, Hebert, & Peterson, 1991). As one physician-anthropologist translates this attitude, "The fear of being sued punishes every single U.S. physician. Since the fact is that the quality of the medicine being practiced does not correlate well with the chance of being sued, it follows that every physician must anticipate a legal action" (Konner, 1993, p. 20).

Many physicians and commentators, in fact, argue that defensive medical practices are less a result of bad legal rules than a product of extreme uncertainty and ambiguity about the precise standard of care against which the practitioner will be judged retrospectively by others (Schopp, 1991). The rules appear to float freely, an especially annoying phenomenon to medical professionals who have been taught to analyze the universe "in terms of yes/no answers" in order "to fix the problem" immediately at hand. Legal scholar Daniel Shuman (1993) has observed:

> The absence of certainty in tort law imposes costs that society is ill-equipped to bear. To ensure that tort law deters unreasonable behavior, the standard of behavior must be communicated to decisionmakers. . . . Although positive law, statutes and administrative rules, inform a portion of tort law, in most negligence trials the jury's determination of reasonableness under the facts and circumstances of an individual case explains the result. No formal system exists to communicate these decisions to the public. Most [nonlegal] lay decisionmakers [including physicians and other health care professionals] learn of these decisions by happenstance, if at all. (p. 125)

In such an environment, physicians for the most part do not fear legal repercussions for violating the law (i.e., practicing below acceptable professional standards). Instead, and much more ominously for the quality of patient care, they are afraid of being drawn involuntarily into the arbitrary and capricious legal process *whether or not* they follow appropriate standards, merely because they and the institutions and organizations within which they deliver care usually happen to be the deepest financial pockets available to "finance the annuities that will assure our patients' future lifestyles." As a gynecologist once told me, "No matter what we [physicians] do, the legal system will screw us." Other physicians frequently intone versions of "Any bad result is a potential liability suit" and simply "I will be sued." Still others bemoan that the tort system targets physicians based on their personalities rather than abilities (Hickson, Clayton, Entman, Miller, Githens, Whetten-Goldstein, et al., 1994, p. 1588).

This way of approaching the world helps account for physicians' almost zero tolerance for personal legal risk. As explained by an attorney who has been a leading critic of unnecessary legal regulation: "But doctors aren't irrational. They're scared because they believe the system is random. Most people don't like to play Russian roulette, even if the odds of getting the bullet are only one in 200. Those are the odds of a test pilot, not a caregiver." (Howard, 1996, p. 58)

Ironically, this attitude—whether right on target or cockeyed—rationally ought to be very liberating in effect, freeing physicians to do whatever they believe is ethically proper rather than concentrating on defensive practices that are thought to be ineffectual anyway. It rarely has this liberating effect, however, as the next chapter's outline of defensive practices illustrates.

GOT A PROBLEM WITH THAT? WHY PHYSICIANS DON'T WANT TO BE SUED

As the previous section explains, most physicians live in constant apprehension of being named a defendant in a medical malpractice lawsuit. There are several important reasons that physicians, although quasi-resigned to that chronic state of jeopardy, try to conduct their practices in ways that they believe can help them avoid or minimize the legal dangers in their midst.

First, and most obvious, there are financial concerns (U.S. Congress, 1994, pp. 27–29). The professional liability insurance that any sane physician carries today, either personally or through an employer, will indemnify or pay the defendant back for any pecuniary (measurable out-of-pocket) and nonpecuniary (pain and suffering) compensatory damages awarded to the plaintiff. Nonetheless, physicians worry that damages will exceed their policy coverage limits, that punitive or exemplary damages that insurance does not cover will be awarded by a runaway jury and jealous judge, and that their future premium payments to purchase insurance coverage will rise steeply if they can even find a company still willing to sell them a policy at any price. More realistically, physicians are concerned about the incidental expenses of defending a lawsuit that insurance does not reimburse, including time lost from practice in consulting with attorneys, reviewing and producing records, undergoing depositions, and attending the trial (Weiler, Hiatt, Newhouse, Johnson, Brennan, & Leape, 1993, pp. 115, 126). Further, there often is anxiety that adverse publicity, even if untrue and later overridden by positive press notices, may scare impressionable patients away from the physician's office.

These financial concerns, however, are definitely secondary for most physicians. The primary toll that a malpractice lawsuit extracts from a physician defendant is, by far, an emotional one.

Attorneys are always advising physicians who are threatened or sued for professional negligence not to "take it personally." Members of the legal profession quickly learn to develop a thick (arguably too thick, in many cases) emotional skin. Members of the medical profession do not, and it is understandable when they reject attorneys' advice on this score and interpret a patient or family's action in bringing a malpractice claim as the *most* personal sort of assault imaginable (Anderson, 1996, p. 15). A lawsuit is particularly and uniquely offensive to physicians, and the vehemence of their negative reaction to the experience far exceeds that of any other kind of professional defendant (Hubbard, 1989, p. 348). Although mainly routine legal boilerplate, terms in legal complaints such as negligent, reckless, careless, unskilled, unfaithful, and unprofessional are difficult for the named physician to keep in perspective (Berczeller, 1994, p. 211). For most of them, there is no emotional distinction between professional and personal competence (even when they grasp the dichotomy intellectually), and public accountability is equated with an attack on the physician's private being (Good, 1995). The physician sees a reputation for not only professional and personal competence at stake but for his or her integrity as well.

Hence, a paradox emerges. Even though physicians join the public in realizing that malpractice cases are an everyday part of contemporary life and that many claims are unsustainable if not absolutely frivolous from their inception, those same physicians nonetheless ordinarily interpret claims brought against themselves as "emotional battles that acquire moral overtones" (Brennan & Berwick, 1996, p. 199). Many physicians describe the experience as a "morality play." A Jewish psychiatrist told me that being sued by a client was a "shanda," or source of great shame. Others use terms such as "embarrassment," "public humiliation," and "bad mark on my moral record."

This overlay of emotional distress (Levinson, 1994, p. 1619) helps to explain why (as noted near the beginning of this chapter) few physicians distinguish between being sued for malpractice, being sued successfully, and being sued rightly. It is the foreign, unfair, often lengthy and full-of-surprises legal process itself that counts emotionally. Even a successful defense is interpreted as "always a Pyhrric victory" (Konner, 1993, p. 20). This is why, for example, even the most well-documented positive reviews of how juries actually perform in medical malpractice cases (Vidmar, 1995) do little to sway physicians' negative attitudes toward the system; if they win (which is the ordinary outcome), physicians still feel they have been put through an emotional hell to get to the point of proving their innocence (Weiler, Hiatt, Newhouse, Johnson, Brennan, & Leape, 1993, p. 75).

All the same, however, the existence of the National Practitioner Data Bank (NPDB) makes all physicians want to be able to escape from a malpractice claim without paying any damages because of a judgment on the claim's merit or a settlement among the parties. Created in the late 1980s by Public Laws 99-660 and 100-93 as part of the Health Care Quality Improvement Act (HCQIA) and implemented in 1990 (45 Code of Federal Regulations § 60), the NPDB keeps records of various penalties imposed on specific physicians and other health care professionals for violations of professional competence or ethics. These violations include medical malpractice payments, adverse licensure actions, adverse actions on clinical privileges by institutions and organizations, and adverse actions on professional society memberships. Hospitals, managed care organizations, other health care entities, medical societies, and insurance companies must submit reports identifying themselves as the reporting entity and the involved medical practitioners. They also must provide descriptive information on the adverse action taken or malpractice payment made.

But the litigation process itself is what remains at the center of physicians' nightmares. Few physicians would vigorously dispute one physician's description of a malpractice trial as "an exercise in character assassination" that provides a forum for our "scapegoating society" to focus on blaming the physician rather than correcting the mistake. There is a widespread belief that any physician's practices can be faulted if dissected after-the-fact under the microscope of expert witnesses and cross-examination by sharp attorneys. Pressures brought on the physician by the liability insurance carrier to settle a case for financial reasons cannot help but exacerbate the situation.

The emotional caldron thus created has bad consequences. Although we must always be exceedingly skeptical about the accuracy of physician self-reports (Peters, Nord, & Woodson, 1986), we cannot responsibly overlook the fact that substantial percentages of sued physicians report impairment of self-esteem and symptoms of clinical depression, anger, fatigue, or irritability (Charles, Wilbert, & Franke, 1985; Charles, Wilbert, & Kennedy, 1984). The stress may be as bad for exonerated defendants as those found guilty of negligently inflicting patient injury (Charles & Kennedy, 1985). There appears to be some evidence that this stress may be severe enough that, for some physicians, the experience of involuntary participation in the legal process by itself makes them so dysfunctional that it predisposes them to being sued again shortly thereafter (Skelly, 1994).

Additionally, the sustained psychological stress of a lawsuit dragging on may lead in some individuals to manifestations of physical illness (Davey, 1990, p. 210). These may include gain or loss of weight, gastrointestinal illnesses, coronary occlusion, and even rare suicides. Weiner and Wettstein (1993, pp. 185–186) liken this "malpractice stress syndrome" to the posttraumatic stress disorder that may follow other life event tensions that take a long time to resolve. A physician who had recently been through the wringer (and who had emerged legally "victorious") lectured me that her unwanted civics lesson was a "debilitating" experience filling her with "outrage" and "resentment."

PARANOIA, REALISTIC FEARS, OR BOTH?

Popular physician perceptions of the risk of ending up as a medical malpractice defendant have a foundation in fact (Sloan, Whetten-Goldstein, Githens, & Entman, 1995, p. 711). Although specific risks vary enormously from medical specialty to specialty and from one geographic area to another, the physician who told me, "There's a lot of litigation against physicians out there" was quite correct. Malpractice claims are filed on a daily basis, accompanied often by substantial publicity, and large financial judgments and settlements occur regularly. Payouts in five of 1995's top ten medical malpractice cases nationally ranged from $40 million to $98.5 million.

That acknowledgement notwithstanding, reliable data about lawsuits—medical malpractice and otherwise—are very scarce (Jacobs, 1995). We really know quite little on the national level about what kinds of cases are brought, which of them go to trial, who wins, how often juries award compensatory and punitive damages, or how much plaintiffs receive in cases settled before trial or during appeal. Some studies suggest that malpractice claims remain relatively rare in the life of an average physician (Bovbjerg & Petronis, 1994, pp. 1424–1425), and that physicians as a group vastly (by at least a factor of three) overestimate the risk that they or their colleagues will be sued (Weiler, Hiatt, Newhouse, Johnson, Brennan, & Leape, 1993, pp. 124–126; Lawthers, Localio, Laird, Lipsitz, Hebert, & Brennan, 1992). Not surprisingly, physicians who have been sued already tend to exaggerate their future risks even more than their nonsued colleagues (Peters, Nord, & Woodson, 1986, p. 611). Even getting physicians to understand intellectually the gulf between their perceptions and the actual liability risks does little to affect their attitudes; after all, I have been told, "One instance is all you need."

Moreover, physicians' ideas about what practice factors predispose them to lawsuits often are wrong or even diametrically opposed to reality. It thus makes sense that "Much of defensive medicine, as currently practiced, may not be effective risk management" (Harris, 1987, p. 2801). For instance, physician beliefs that they are at highest legal risk for sharing too much correct, relevant information with a patient or for acknowledging to the patient that the physician does not know the answer to a particular question are as substantively erroneous as they are pervasively held (Rosoff, 1994, p. 315). Similarly, most physicians' faulty but sure conception of the legal standards used to adjudicate malpractice cases (Liang, 1996) reminds one of the old, unintentionally ironic refrain, "I may not be correct, but at least I'm not in doubt."

Thus, physicians should tread cautiously in formulating opinions and attitudes about their legal environment and how they should strategically deal with it. In practice, the exact opposite usually occurs, with those opinions and attitudes more frequently taking the shape of "figment[s] of excited brains" (Cardozo, 1921, p. 122) than of accurate, dispassionate evaluations of reality. The vast majority of physicians with whom I regularly converse confidently lecture attorneys and their peers on the substantive legal rules that affect their medical practices (Greenlaw, 1994, p. 554), freely employing absolute terms such as "never," "always," and "must." The natural, but rarely posed, inquiry arising from this emphatic "I know what the law says and it's bad" sort of behavior (which, not incidentally, stands in stark paradoxical contrast to physicians' complaints about the law's ambiguity in setting and communicating standards of care) is: What is the etiology of physician perceptions, and more importantly misperceptions, about the law?

THE ORIGIN OF SPECIOUS IDEAS (AND SOME VALID ONES, TOO)

To get directly to the point, where do physicians come up with their ideas about what the law requires of, permits, and forbids them? When I asked one physician this question, he responded profoundly, "God knows!" The more useful answer is considerably more complex, multifaceted, and problematic (Greenlaw, 1994, p. 554): from risk managers and in-house legal counsel (see Chapter 3), each other, medical leaders and role models who pontificate both general and specific war stories, throwaway publications and media spots, the professional educational process, drug companies, and insurers and other vendors of risk management services and products. Given this constellation of informational sources, there should be little wonder that folklore, anecdotes, and stereotypes usually triumph.

Undoubtedly the most powerful source of (mis)information (McCrary, Swanson, Perkins, & Winslade, 1992, at 371) about the law for most physicians is "the medical grapevine" or "physician sob session"—that is, the constant stream of informal conversations on this topic they carry on with their physician peers in the hospital locker room, lounge, and cafeteria and at medical society dinners. "Physicians listen to other physicians." This "oral tradition" that flows from the "medical culture" ordinarily revolves around personal anecdotes; most physicians prefer concrete cases to abstract theories. If bloody enough and entertainingly rendered, a single anecdote can cause otherwise scientifically minded physicians (who spend a lot of time trying to put clinical risks into realistic perspective for their patients) to grossly overestimate their own risk of litigation, just as laypersons inevitably blow out of realistic proportion their personal risk of dying in an airplane crash upon hearing about a tragic but isolated aviation accident.

The most gripping tales are told by physician colleagues who have returned from the near-death experience of a "legal episode"—that is, being threatened or sued personally. Many physicians with such personal experience purposely maintain a low profile among their peers; they have been counseled to keep quiet while their case is pending and just want to put the incident behind them after it has been resolved. Those who choose to describe their crucifixion and resurrection to other physicians, however, often take on the status of folk hero and instant expert, with few of their peers willing to challenge the claims of the legally baptized that "Doing X got me into trouble," or conversely, "saved my hide" and "You won't believe what I am going through, what records I am being told to produce, and what conduct I am being forced to justify."

The other main version of physician-to-physician communication about the legal shadow darkening the glow of medical practice consists of fifth-hand, unsubstantiated hearsay—for example, "A friend of a friend told X to Jim, and this is what I overheard him telling Mary about how that physician got into trouble." Often the stories begin with a real incident, but (like the old party game "telephone") distortion sets in by the time that partial, inaccurate, and embellished retelling upon retelling has converted the occurrence into a "legend."

In both kinds of verbal interchanges, spreading word-of-mouth "popular wisdom," the storyteller and listener alike routinely engage unconsciously in selective telling and hearing, with the most anxiety-provoking parts of the story receiving greatest attention. Only the "most frightful" of these "urban myths" get repeated and remembered under this fragmented approach to information dissemination, the gossip and rumors of quick "curbside consultations" leading to conclusions without facts (Meisel & Kuczewski, 1996). One physician likens this process to the way that people several years ago were convinced to believe (wrongly) that alligators lived in the New York City sewer system and might enter an apartment through the toilet bowl. "One bad case travels like wildfire," and adverse legal outcomes thus exert a chilling influence on medical practice far out of proportion to their likelihood of occurrence, but physicians seldom "waste" each others' time discussing the much larger number of potentially volatile patient care situations that are worked out satisfactorily. Even if the latter cases were included in the discussion, one unsubstantiated remark about "knowing someone who got into trouble doing that" would quickly negate any constructive lessons.

Distinct from, but related to, the peer-to-peer oral tradition of "infinite intellectual regress" regarding legal issues is the power of pontification by professional leaders and role models who do not grasp the significance of their encyclicals. Ignorant mentors are especially dangerous because they are treated as authority figures despite their ignorance. Inflamed attitudes cannot help but be inculcated when, for example, new physicians at a major university are told by their honored graduation speaker:

> Unfortunately, there is a profession that thrives on the untoward outcomes in medical practice, the legal profession. Operating on a contingency-fee basis, lawyers swarm like biting flies around our heads. . . . Too often the result is a frivolous suit, settled quietly to avoid physician embarrassment. And sometimes the awards made by a sympathetic jury are absolutely astonishing. (Neel, 1994, p. 21)

After informal peer gossip and inflammatory leadership pronouncements, the most important food source for skewed legal imaginations for most clinicians is the mass of throwaway publications and other media tidbits that threaten to overwhelm the medical mail recipient literally every day. The limited medicolegal reading time of most physicians, particularly those who are engaged in full-time clinical practice as opposed to teaching and research, is devoted almost exclusively to sensationalized, eye-catching news blurbs and short essays in non-refereed, tabloid-style newspapers and magazines (Greenlaw, 1994, p. 554) that usually are given away free to anyone with a license to prescribe the drugs that are advertised therein. Such "medicolegal lite" may be published by commercial ventures or professional trade associations.

These brief written sound bites, with tremendous potential for inspiring knee-jerk defensive responses, rarely describe underlying facts or arguments in sufficient depth to permit intelligent reflection. Few of the "journalists" churning out this verbiage possess any meaningful educational or practical background concerning the issues upon which they are holding forth, but they all have learned well how to depict the most unusual and idiosyncratic medicolegal situations—those which have the least to profitably teach practitioners—as though they were typical albeit appalling cases.

To the extent that physicians watch television and listen to radio, the reports in these media forms are equally distressing. Presentations about medical malpractice broadcast in these outlets generally mimic the titillating *National Inquirer*–style approach that has proven so popular in the trade print media. Only the most sensational and distorted stories are likely to earn airtime.

As one physician confided to me, "A news clip that spends 30 seconds focusing on outrageous and exceptional results sticks with physicians who see it for years. Physicians talk forever about the case where such and such happened. Notorious exceptions are not seen as the exceptions they are, but rather as the invariable rule from that day forward." One observer has written, "In malpractice law, a single frightening case has surprising *de facto* power," feeding a vicious cycle in which physician practices may change sufficiently in response to perceptions about that outlier case to actually alter the standard of care to reflect those changed practices (Morreim, 1994, p. 87). To compound the problem, by the time an outlandish malpractice judgment awarded in a malpractice lawsuit and reported as the lead story of the day is (as happens regularly) eventually reversed or reduced, that case somehow always loses its lead story appeal.

Perhaps even more instructive is identifying those potential information and analysis sources that virtually never actually inform physicians' thinking about malpractice issues, namely, serious scholarly articles published in respected, peer-reviewed medical and health care journals. The major peer-reviewed journals, like the *New England Journal of Medicine* and the *Journal of the American Medical Association*, regularly provide forums for well-written, comprehensively researched pieces that analyze significant topics related to medical malpractice in a thoughtful and dispassionate manner. The problem is that, except for those employed full-time in academic settings who usually peruse at least the abstracts in leading journals, physicians fail to read precisely those contributions to the literature from which they might derive the most useful insight.

Surely, the physician who told me, "Physicians do all of their reading on the toilet, so anything more than one page doesn't stand a chance," had to be overstating the point. However, few full-time medical practitioners admit to doing more than scanning the tables of contents of the major journals and perhaps reading the abstract or even occasional entire article in their particular specialty journal if, but only if, the article has direct, immediate (i.e., right now) significance for their own practice. Moreover, when a bona fide article is merely scanned rather than studied by physicians, the stage is set for misinterpretation and miscitation of the author's proposed message.

Some practitioners would like to read thoroughly and reflect in depth upon more articles, including those with medicolegal content, published in the respectable journals, but are forced by the crush of time constraints to be highly selective. For many, though, time pressures are a secondary consideration; the majority of physicians probably avoid reading scholarly medicolegal analyses in the leading national journals precisely because they are scholarly, preferring instead to get their quasi-information from terse, intellectually unadorned and unchallenging, concretely case-based snippets in medical tabloids. Physicians generally are scared away from reading, let alone working at understanding and making practice adaptations based on, scholarly articles that appear to be more "a rich gourmet meal rather than a good fast food hamburger." Moreover, in the medicolegal realm many physicians cannot tell the difference between printed junk and substantive discussion in the literature and thus put undue credence on the former. A number of physicians call their accountants and attorneys after reading throwaway articles and arrive at financial and perceived risk management decisions in response to that written hysteria. Indeed, it is the sensational tone of the tabloids that makes them both more interesting and more credible to most physicians than the stolid academic prose and dull, evenhanded exegeses of the serious journals. The reverse snobbery of full-time practitioners is as instructive as it is dismaying. Reacting to an article suggesting that physicians should actually have a valid reason before ordering ankle X rays, one physician who has the answers tells readers: "Only some disconnected academic who is not performing grunt orthopedics on the street would recommend taking no ankle X rays. Most of the rest of us are going to continue to take them. We know we don't need them, but you have to prove it in court" (Hale, 1995).

Another thing that physicians practically never read is the law itself, even when it is handed to them. Many state and local medical associations have put together booklets reprinting the language of relevant federal and state statutes for their members, but it is likely that these booklets go largely unread by the medical infantry. Similarly, the percentage of physicians who have actually read any of the judicial decisions to which they constantly and confidently refer in their conversations probably hovers in the low single figures. This is no doubt one of the reasons that advice to physicians not to worry so much about legal entanglements (Annas, 1995) invariably falls on deaf ears; physicians see the world through the lens of the tabloids, not that of appellate judges, legislators, or—heaven forbid—law professors.

Despite the distressing discussion to this point, scholarly contributions to the legitimate medical literature and compilations of the law itself on medical malpractice topics serve a valuable purpose even though they are generally ignored, if not actively shunned, by the rank and file of clinical medicine. Many members of medicine's "elites"—for example, educators, medical staff leaders, institutional ethics committee and institutional review board members, and officers in major professional associations—do read the pertinent law and at least a portion of this literature and sometimes even are influenced in their thinking and conduct by the substantive medicolegal explanations these peer-reviewed articles contain. These elites, in turn, may be in a direct or indirect position to create a positive ripple or trickle-down effect by using their understanding to influence changes in the policies and procedures of health care institutions and organizations and, ultimately, in the practices of individual physicians.

The fact that something on a legal topic appears in a respected medical journal, of course, in no way assures that it is accurate or instructive in a positive sense. For instance, the harm done by the grossly misinformed assertion, "Many malpractice suits have resulted from withdrawing life support, even when legal documents clearly expressed the patient's wishes to have life support discontinued" (Reich, 1997), is probably multiplied several-fold precisely because it appears legitimated by virtue of publication in a prestigious venue. When hysterical misinformation appears not only in a respected publication, but under the authorship of a physician deemed by peers preeminent in his or her clinical specialty, the damage is difficult to contain. Many physicians will accept at face value, no doubt, heart surgeon Denton Cooley's (1997, p. 13) outlandish comparison of the "good old days" of medical practice with the awful present, "Today, malpractice suits, unheard of in the early part of the century [sic], are common occurrences, and physicians must carry insurance to protect themselves against the inevitable [sic] judgment," based on the demonstrably wrong assumption that great skill in the technical aspects of medicine also confers special competence and wisdom regarding its social facets.

The formal educational process through which every physician must travel is not a particularly positive source of medicolegal understanding and appreciation for many of its participants. Although most medical schools think that they are teaching something about liability to their students, good curricula and—much more importantly—competent instruction in this area are scarce (Hamilton, 1991).

That absence does not at all mean that legal, especially malpractice, issues go unmentioned in the classroom or its clinical equivalent. On the contrary, at the medical student level, clinical instructors as well as fellow students and residents with no formal education in legal matters do not let that little deficiency keep them from freely sharing their definitively pronounced legal insights. Such indoctrination from one generation to another in many respects is one of the rites of passage that students are expected to internalize on their way to full membership in the medical culture. Because mentors have power over careers, students assume them to be as authoritative regarding legal matters as in areas where the mentors really do have expertise—particularly if the mentor can tell personal war stories about fighting the legal system.

If the students are lucky—very lucky—there might be a knowledge-able faculty member around to repair the informational damage inflicted by others. In an article praising the efforts of one medical school to integrate the organized study of moral complexities into the undergraduate medical curriculum, one student instructs his receptive peers to falsify records: "I understand why you do it. A skillful lawyer could come back and make it look like something was brewing and you let it go. So you pad it [the patient's medical record] a little bit." Fortunately, a professor with judgment as well as some legal knowledge was immediately available to caution the students not to buy thoughtlessly into the myths that are rampant in health settings about why physicians lose malpractice cases (Shea, 1996, p. A40), but such availability is rare.

Damage can also be inflicted when a medical school thinks that it has done its legal education job by bringing in a local litigation attorney periodically to entertain students with embellished tales that reinforce all of the bad stereotypes about the legal system with which the students have begun their medical careers. From the outset, the message conveyed about law and lawyers is "Stay away."

It is at the residency-training level that inculcation of litigation and liability fears really shifts into high gear. An Office of Technology Assessment study concluded:

> Young physicians in residency training may be particularly susceptible to learning defensive practices—either explictly or implicitly—from their supervisors and faculty. Graduate medical education may thus help perpetuate defensive medicine at both the conscious and unconscious levels. (U.S. Congress, 1994, p. 37)

Specific postgraduate training programs, varying widely by specialty, may include a smattering of formal instruction about legal issues. However, residents learn about defensive medicine primarily by observing the behavior of attending physicians and more-senior residents and talking with them about problems (legal issues always being posed in a negative light) identified in the context of particular patients. In essence, physicians-in-training learn about law in the identical manner they learn about medicine—namely, by following around physicians, who often are only a step or two ahead of them in the training process, and imitating their conduct. When teachers complain about the malpractice climate and react defensively to it, those whom they are teaching are taught to mimic that attitude and reaction. Myths about the law do not get dispelled, because junior participants in the educational process either do not know enough or are afraid to challenge their medical elders, and moreover do not feel confident enough or that they have the time to research legal issues independently.

Formal continuing medical education (CME) programs, including those contained within professional organizational meetings, sometimes perpetuate legal misperceptions for physicians engaged in practice. The skewing of CME presentations in the direction of legal hysteria is attributable to several factors. Certainly, most erroneously biased CME presentations are given by physicians or others who sincerely believe in the accuracy of the misinformation they are perpetuating. A very significant aspect is the fact that many CME programs are supported financially by pharmaceutical companies. Although current ethical guidelines prohibit commercial sponsors from directly selecting CME program speakers or content (Kapp, 1992), a sponsor's influence may be observed in numerous indirect ways. Thus, it is not unusual for a speaker at a CME to inform the physician audience, "Prescribe X drug or you are committing malpractice (and will be sued for all your present and future income and possessions). X is the standard of care," where X happens to be a drug marketed by the program sponsor.

This problem is not limited to physician CME presenters. The *Wall Street Journal* (King, 1995, p. A4) reported on a malpractice attorney whose speaking fee was paid by Genentech Inc. to warn physicians at a series of CME programs that the public expects one of Genentech's products (TPA) to be used in heart attack victims whether or not it is superior to rival drugs and despite its steep price, and will sue if those expectations are disappointed.

Even scientifically sound, objectively presented CME programs may have negative repercussions in terms of the legal lessons drawn by physician attendees. Some physicians claim that attending these kinds of programs tends to increase their nervousness about liability exposure, because speakers ordinarily are experts on the cutting edge of their respective fields and therefore intentionally or inadvertently frighten the audience by emphasizing what latest developments most full-time clinicians do not know much about or regularly incorporate into their care of patients. In an environment characterized by increasing competition for CME program attendees, there is a need to market programs as presenting the absolutely current state of the art based upon the most recent data. This showcasing of what is thought at that particular moment to be optimal treatment in many instances encourages excessive medical intervention by making practitioners uneasily overreact to their own previous informational and practice deficiencies.

The role of formal risk management initiatives concerning defensive medicine and patient care is discussed in detail in Chapter 3. Suffice it to mention here, as part of this discussion of the etiology of physicians' ideas about the legal jungle waiting to pounce on their every miscue, that physicians are barraged daily by mail and telephone, by advertisements and other sales entreaties, by vendors of risk management products such as publications, tapes, personalized risk management audits, and seminars. Typical is the letter sent to all American psychiatrists dated August 24, 1994, from Psychiatric Times, advertising an upcoming CME program with the admonition:

> Coming on the heels of managed care carve outs, cutbacks, gatekeepers and prospective reviews to treat our patients, it [a recent highly publicized, controversial case in which a psychiatrist was found liable for $500,000 to a former patient's father] may seem almost too much to bear. **Some lawyers are calling for mandatory informed consent for psychotherapy and even disclosure to prospective patients of our treatment outcomes with former patients.** I kid you not!
>
> The hassles and the spotlight of public scrutiny from these controversial issues will not go away because they are regrettable. **We are under siege in America in 1994. Protect your career!** (bold type in original)

Liability insurance carriers also market their policies by portraying physicians' personal risk exposure as expansively as possible. Risk management and insurance advertisements join, along with the sensationalist print and electronic media noted previously that continuously assault physicians, to exert a synergistically negative effect on their audience's psyche.

STRIKING A NERVE: PHYSICIANS AS THEIR OWN WORST CRITICS

Physician antipathy toward the legal system may be as deep and intense as it is because this mode of external scrutiny underscores and reinforces many of the frustrations and self-doubts that physicians themselves harbor about their own performance. Physicians are usually their own most demanding critics and resent outsiders publicly rubbing in medical shortcomings and limitations. Because they answer to their consciences and their peers, few physicians feel that they should also have to answer to others.

Tort standards require that physicians provide reasonable care under the circumstances. By contrast, physicians expect a higher standard of themselves: perfection (Snyder & Brennan, 1996, p. 51). They are socialized into a "culture of infallibility" (Levy, 1995, p. 39), in which errors in patient care are not about training or technique. Instead, errors are manifestations of unacceptable character flaws, and being accused in a public forum of committing an error by an external scrutinizer cannot be interpreted other than as a personal affront (Leape, 1994, p. 1851). One physician has summed up this orientation:

> Upon being served with a summons, the initial reaction is one of be-numbed disbelief followed by self-deprecating analysis, schooled as the physician is in the pursuit of excellence, then feelings of inadequacy, and, finally, anger, frustration, and a tremendous sense of isolation. (Davey, 1990, p. 210)

"In a profession that values perfection, error is virtually forbidden," comments the author of a study of the emotional impact of mistakes made by physicians (Newman, 1996). Speaking about a serious patient care error he had made, one family practitioner participating in that study remarked, "So I closed off the issue and just tacked it away. Ultimately medicine tends to drive us away from our feelings and from getting close to the people. That behavior makes it hard for us doctors to come together."

Furthermore, physicians ordinarily do a much worse job than juries or judges in distinguishing between honest and negligent errors, often blurring blameworthy deviation from acceptable professional stan-dards and blameless misfortune (Bosk, 1979, p. 24). Even when they would not be held to be at fault legally, physicians tend to envision themselves as lifeguards upon whose shift no one should be allowed to drown. Compliance with scientific evidence and reasoning rarely as-suages the physician's guilt feelings induced by a disastrous clinical result or the embarassment ("losing face") occasioned when such a result is called to the attention of one's professional peers.

Physicians can never be immunized against their own feelings; pro-fessionalism does not mean a suspension of emotions and self-doubt. With or without the added pressures of legal system intrusion, errors associated with seriously bad patient outcomes are "etched indelibly" in the physician's mind (Bosk, 1979, p. 40). Some physicians make mistakes from which they never fully recover emotionally, and almost all go through some sense of introspection amounting to psychological torment in rehashing the error multiple times within their own minds (Hart, 1995; Wu, Folkman, McPhee, & Lo, 1993). They take bad out-comes to heart and crave a reaffirmation of personal competence (Good, 1995; Berczeller, 1994, pp. 216–217; Hilfiker, 1984), the right to be able to sleep well at night again.

Both physicians and patients are harmed when physicians attempt to hide their errors (whether negligent or blameless) from patients, medi-cal colleagues, and other third parties. They blame this defensive prac-tice on the fear that they will suffer legal and/or financial punishments if they do otherwise. This form of defensive practice is explored further in Chapter 2. In Chapter 7, possible public policy interventions to deal more effectively with the errors-in-medicine problem by alleviating some of the claimed legal anxieties are outlined.

Closely connected to the problem of medical errors is the substantial difficulty that most physicians experience in dealing with the concepts of medical and legal uncertainty. In every case, "Medical decision making is a probabilistic enterprise," and often decisions must be made and acted upon before the uncertainty can be resolved or even appreciably reduced (Bosk, 1979, p. 23). Physicians, socialized to expect perfection and wanting to believe that problems all have dichotomous right/wrong answers that they could know if they only had enough information, generally react poorly to the real world of medical gray areas and information voids (Logan & Scott, 1996; Gerrity, Earp, DeVellis, & Light, 1992; Gerrity, DeVellis, & Earp, 1990).

Similarly, physicians are frustrated because the law, particularly in the malpractice arena with its multiple sources and constant evolution of standards, is often uncertain and ambiguous at any discrete point in time. Physicians want an impossible degree of prospective certainty from the legal system in every conceivable set of circumstances, and they tolerate the gap between expectation and performance poorly (Morreim, 1990). In the next chapter, I suggest that a fair amount of defensive medical practice that is blamed on fear of litigation and liability is really driven by physicians' uneasy and not always peaceful coexistence with the medical and legal uncertainty that they constantly confront.

CONCLUSION

This chapter has outlined briefly how physicians generally perceive their legal risks within the current medical malpractice environment that engulfs them, as well as physician attitudes toward law and the legal system more broadly. Many of the perceptions commonly held in this sphere are questionable and even outright erroneous. Nonetheless, perceived legal constraints have always been a much more important force than the truth in shaping actual physician behavior toward patients (McCrary, Swanson, Perkins, & Winslade, 1992, p. 374). It is to the subject of physician behavior, so motivated and influenced, that I turn in the next chapter.

NOTES

1. Accordingly, this chapter concentrates on civil tort lawsuits alleging medical malpractice brought against individual physicians and other health care profession-

als and organizations by individual patients or their families. Anxieties about potential criminal and civil regulatory scrutiny and punishment are discussed chiefly in Chapters 5 and 6.

REFERENCES

Anderson, E. (1996, March 4). Physician won malpractice case, but still lost a lot. *American Medical News, 39*, 15–16.

Annas, G. J. (1996). Facilitating choice: Judging the physician's role in abortion and suicide. *Quinnipiac Health Law Journal, 1*, 93–112.

Annas, G. J. (1995). Medicine, death, and the criminal law. *New England Journal of Medicine, 333*, 527–530.

Berczeller, P. H. (1994). *Doctors and patients: What we feel about you.* New York: Macmillan Publishing Company.

Bosk, C. L. (1979). *Forgive and remember: Managing medical failure.* Chicago: University of Chicago Press.

Bovbjerg, R. R., & Petronis, K. R. (1994). The relationship between physicians' malpractice claims history and later claims: Does the past predict the future? *Journal of the American Medical Association, 272*, 1421–1426.

Brennan, T. A., & Berwick, D. M. (1996). *New rules: Regulation, markets, and the quality of American health care.* San Francisco: Jossey-Bass.

Brennan, T. A., Sox, C. M., & Burstin, H. R. (1996). Relation between negligent adverse events and the outcomes of medical-malpractice litigation. *New England Journal of Medicine, 335*, 1963–1967.

Britten, N. (1995). Patients' demands for prescriptions in primary care. *British Medical Journal, 310*, 1084–1085.

Cardozo, B. L. (1921). *The nature of the judicial process.* New Haven: Yale University Press.

Charles, S. C., & Kennedy, E. (1985). *Defendant: A psychiatrist on trial for medical malpractice.* New York: Free Press.

Charles, S. C., Wilbert, J. R., & Franke, K. J. (1985). Sued and nonsued physicians' self-reported reactions to malpractice litigation. *American Journal of Psychiatry, 142*, 437–440.

Charles, S. C., Wilbert, J. R., & Kennedy, E. C. (1984). Physicians' self-reports of reactions to malpractice litigation. *American Journal of Psychiatry, 141*, 563–565.

Cooley, D. A. (1997). Medical practice: Past, present, future. *Pharos, 60*(1), 13–16.

Davey, L. M. (1990). The hidden costs of malpractice. *Connecticut Medicine, 54*, 209–211.

Ferguson, E. F., Jr. (1993). For legal reasons. *Journal of the Florida Medical Association, 80*, 61–62.

Gerrity, M. S., DeVellis, R. F., & Earp, J. (1990). Physicians' reactions to uncertainty in patient care: A new measure and new insights. *Medical Care, 28*, 724–736.

Gerrity, M. S., Earp, J. L., DeVellis, R. F., & Light, D. W. (1992). Uncertainty and professional work: Perceptions of physicians in clinical practice. *American Journal of Sociology, 97*, 1022–1051.

Good, M.-J. D. (1995). *American medicine: The quest for competence.* Berkeley, CA: University of California Press.

Greenlaw, J. (1994). Introductory remarks to a symposium on the legal and ethical implications of innovative medical technology. *Albany Law Review,* 57, 551–558.

Hale, W. R. (1995, November). Lawyers make ankle X-rays necessary [Letter] *Johns Hopkins Magazine, 47,* 8.

Hamilton, T. E. (1991). How issues of professional liability are taught in U.S. medical schools. *Academic Medicine, 66,* 39–40.

Harris, J. E. (1987). Defensive medicine: It costs, but does it work? *Journal of the American Medical Association, 257,* 2801–2802.

Hart, R. G. (1995). Lost sleep. *Annals of Emergency Medicine, 25,* 849–850.

Hickson, G. B., Clayton, E. W., Entman, S. S., Miller, C. S., Githens, P. B., Whetten-Goldstein, K., et al. (1994). Obstetricians' prior malpractice experience and patients' satisfaction with care. *Journal of the American Medical Association, 272,* 1583–1587.

Hilfiker, D. (1984). Facing our mistakes. *New England Journal of Medicine, 310,* 118–122.

Howard, P. K. (1996, March). Book review of *Medical Malpractice and the American Jury* by N. Vidmar. *Washington Monthly, 28,* 55–58.

Hubbard, F. P. (1989). The physicians' point of view concerning medical malpractice: A sociological perspective on the symbolic importance of "tort reform." *Georgia Law Review, 23,* 295–358.

Jacobs, M. A. (1995, June 9). Reliable data about lawsuits are very scarce. *Wall Street Journal,* pp. B1–B2.

Kapp, M. B. (1992). Ethical issues in the relationship between American physicians and drug companies. *International Journal of Risk and Safety in Medicine, 3,* 73–80.

King, R. T., Jr. (1995, January 10). In marketing of drugs, Genentech tests limits of what is acceptable. *Wall Street Journal,* pp. A1, A4.

Konner, M. (1993). *Medicine at the crossroads.* New York: Pantheon Books.

Lawthers, A. G., Localio, A. R., Laird, N. M., Lipsitz, S., Hebert, L., & Brennan, T. A. (1992). Physicians' perceptions of the risk of being sued. *Journal of Health Politics, Policy and Law, 17,* 463–482.

Leape, L. L. (1994). Error in medicine. *Journal of the American Medical Association, 272,* 1851–1857.

Levinson, W. (1994). Physician-patient communication: A key to malpractice prevention. *Journal of the American Medical Association, 272,* 1619–1620.

Levy, R. (1995, Fall). Code blue. *Harvard Public Health Review, 7,* 36–41.

Liang, B. A. (1996). Medical malpractice: Do physicians have knowledge of legal standards and assess cases as juries do? *University of Chicago Law School Roundtable, 3,* 59–111.

Localio, A. R., Lawthers, A. G., Brennan, T. A., Laird, N. M., Hebert, L. E., & Peterson, L. M. (1991). Relation between malpractice claims and adverse events due to negligence. *New England Journal of Medicine, 325,* 245–251.

Logan, R. L., & Scott, P. J. (1996). Uncertainty in clinical practice: Implications for quality and costs of health care. *Lancet, 347,* 595–598.

McCrary, S. V., Swanson, J. W., Perkins, H. S., & Winslade, W. J. (1992). Treatment decisions for terminally ill patients: Physicians' legal defensiveness and knowledge of medical law. *Law, Medicine & Health Care, 20*, 364–376.

McQuade, J. S. (1991). The medical malpractice crisis—reflections on the alleged causes and proposed cures. *Journal of the Royal Society of Medicine, 84*, 408–411.

Meisel, A., & Kuczewski, M. (1996). Legal and ethical myths about informed consent. *Archives of Internal Medicine, 156*, 2521–2526.

Morreim, E. H. (1994). Redefining quality by reassigning responsibility. *American Journal of Law and Medicine, 20*, 79–104.

Morreim, E. H. (1990, Spring). The law of nature and the law of the land. *The Pharos, 53*, 1–6.

Neel, J. V. (1994, Fall). A time of change. *The Pharos, 57*, 19–22.

Newman, M. C. (1996). The emotional impact of mistakes on family physicians. *Archives of Family Medicine, 5*, 71–75.

Peters, J. D., Nord, S. K., & Woodson, R. D. (1986). An empirical analysis of the medical and legal professions' experiences and perceptions of medical and legal malpractice. *University of Michigan Journal of Law Reform, 19*, 601–636.

Reich, J. S. (1997). Letter. *Annals of Internal Medicine, 126*, 587.

Rosoff, A. J. (1994). Truce on the battlefield: A proposal for a different approach to medical informed consent. *Journal of Law, Medicine & Ethics, 22*, 314–317.

Schopp, R. F. (1991). The psychotherapist's duty to protect the public: The appropriate standard and the foundation in legal theory and empirical premises. *Nebraska Law Review, 70*, 327–360.

Shea, C. (1996, May 3). Beyond anatomy class. *Chronicle of Higher Education*, A39–A40.

Shuman, D. W. (1993). The psychology of deterrence in tort law. *Kansas Law Review, 42*, 115–168.

Skelly, F. J. (1994, November 7). Scope of stress. *American Medical News, 37* (17), 20–21.

Sloan, F. A., Whetten-Goldstein, K., Githens, P. B., & Entman, S. S. (1995). Effects of the threat of medical malpractice litigation and other factors on birth outcomes. *Medical Care, 33*, 700–714.

Snyder, L., & Brennan, T. A. (1996). Disclosure of errors and the threat of malpractice. In L. Snyder (Ed.), *Ethical choices: Case studies for medical practice* (pp. 47–52). Philadelphia: American College of Physicians.

Sox, H. C., & Nease, R. F. (1993). When doctor and patient disagree. *Journal of General Internal Medicine, 8*, 580–581.

Tyler, T. R. (1990). *Why people obey the law.* New Haven: Yale University Press.

U.S. Congress, Office of Technology Assessment (1994). *Defensive medicine and medical malpractice.* OTA-H-602. Washington, DC: U.S. Government Printing Office.

Vidmar, N. (1995). *Medical malpractice and the American jury.* Ann Arbor, MI: University of Michigan Press.

Weiler, P. C., Hiatt, H. H., Newhouse, J. P., Johnson, W. G., Brennan, T. A., & Leape, L. L. (1993). *A measure of malpractice: Medical injury, malpractice litigation, and patient compensation.* Cambridge, MA: Harvard University Press.

Weiner, B. A., & Wettstein, R. M. (1993). *Legal issues in mental health care*. New York: Plenum Press.

Williams, P. C., & Winslade, W. (1995). Educating medical students about law and the legal system. *Academic Medicine, 70,* 777–786.

Wolter, T. J. (1993). In the footsteps. *Journal of the American Medical Association, 269,* 2947.

Wright, J. D. (1995). Metaphors and health care reform [Letter]. *New England Journal of Medicine, 333,* 259–260.

Wu, A. W., Folkman, S., McPhee, S. J., & Lo, B. (1993). How house officers cope with their mistakes. *Western Journal of Medicine, 159,* 565–569.

The Lawyer Made Me Do It: From Legal Perception to Medical Practice

As Chapter 1 makes clear, there is a crisis mentality regarding medical malpractice among American physicians at the close of the twentieth century. As attorney Mark Hall (1991, p. 119) has noted, "Although this crisis mentality may result in part from uncritical acceptance of interest group dogma, to the extent that a crisis is in fact widely perceived, it has the quality of a self-fulfilling prophesy: if doctors believe, rightly or wrongly, that malpractice suits are out of control, they will practice more defensively." (The defensive practice virus has recently begun to infect the practice of law, too [Jacobs, 1995], but that is a topic deserving its own volume.)

Physicians almost uniformly perceive the behavior caused by their legal apprehensions as negative on the quality of patient care. Frequent phrases expressing these sentiments are to the effect, "If only I were free to practice medicine without fear of possible litigation, I could do things very differently [i.e., better for my patients]," and "I would treat my spouse differently [i.e., better] than the rest of my patients, because [s]he wouldn't sue me if luck brought a bad result."[1]

Pediatrician Catherine DeAngelis's (1987) sentiments are typical:

Liability insurance to provide recompense to patients and to protect clinicians is both fair and good. However, the reimbursement mechanism must

be based on legal fault and not on personal economics, sympathy, or whim.
Until this can be accomplished, patients, their families, and physicians will
not be treated justly. (p. 880)

There is widespread consensus that the practice of defensive medicine by physicians wary of medical malpractice allegations contributes
to the problem of escalating health care expenditures in the United
States (U.S. Congress, 1993; Greene, Goldberg, Beattie, Russo, Ellison,
& Dalen, 1989; Reynolds, Rizzo, & Gonzalez, 1987). As one national
health policy leader has put it, "There can be no doubt that fear of
litigation drives many physicians to wasteful styles of practice, which,
when added to the ever-increasing premiums for liability insurance,
contribute to the rising costs of health care" (Relman, 1989). Throwing
away reusable medical devices after only one use because of fear of a
lawsuit if problems were to develop on subsequent uses is one obvious
and common example of this waste. The Physician Payment Review
Commission noted in its 1994 Annual Report to Congress, "There is
great concern that liability considerations may hinder efforts to reduce
the delivery of inefficient or ineffective care" (p. 291). Beyond that
general notion, though, there exists widespread and deep disagreement
over a precise working definition of the defensive medicine phenomenon and its magnitude and specific clinical and economic manifestations (Harris, 1987).

"Wasteful" medicine is not completely synonymous with "bad"
medicine, as defined in terms of suboptimal quality and ethical
violations in patient care, but surely the two concepts are connected.
At the least, they fall into overlapping circles on a Venn diagram. If
physicians claim that the defensive medicine that causes waste is a
deviation, induced by a threat of legal repercussions, from what the
physician believes is sound practice and is generally regarded in the
medical community as such (Hershey, 1972), then it is, by definition,
not good medicine.

In this chapter, I critically dissect physicians' claims that the antago-
nistic legal environment within which they toil inspires defensive practices that may harm patients, with special attention to the key ethical
principles of beneficence, nonmaleficence, autonomy, and social or
distributive justice. I particularly concentrate on ways in which defensive medicine: jeopardizes the physician's ability to help or do good for
patients (thereby violating beneficence); makes the physician inflict
potential harm on patients (thwarting nonmaleficence); forces the physician to impinge upon the self-determination or free choice of patients
(thus affronting autonomy); and pressures the physician to act in ways
that unnecessarily impair access to needed medical care, either for

particular patients or regarding particular forms of care (with consequent adverse implications for social or distributive justice).

DEFINING AND MEASURING DEFENSIVE MEDICINE: GOOD REASONS AND REAL REASONS

Physicians take defensive medicine for granted, as a "given" part of their professional lives, often referring to the "lawyer's tax" on care (Evans, 1996, p. 1449) imposed by the perpetual need they feel to look over their shoulders. Despite all the talk, "There is a paucity of empirical evidence on the effect of the threat of a medical malpractice suit on practice patterns. There is virtually no empirical evidence on the effect of the threat on health outcomes" (Sloan, Whetten-Goldstein, Githens, & Entman, 1995, p. 701). "Unfortunately, the rhetoric with regard to defensive medicine has not been matched by good empirical research on the subject. Indeed, there are no reliable studies on defensive medicine, and for good reason" (Brennan, 1991, p. 135). Although we can verify the existence of certain defensive behavior, like purchasing higher coverage limits of liability insurance (Milgrom, Whitney, Conrad, Fiset, & O'Hara, 1995), we do not really know whether, and how, physicians treat their patients differently because of litigation and liability worries.

Although we have acknowledged our ignorance in this area for at least the last several decades (Tancredi & Barondess, 1978), little has been done to remedy it. As physician-attorney Troyen Brennan (1995) explains:

> Empirical investigation of the effect of law on behavior is not highly regarded in legal academe. Law reviews generally report analyses of case law or theoretical underpinnings of litigation. Case books rarely emphasize quantitative analyses. Few faculty conduct research involving specification and proof of hypothesis. This is true on both the right and the left of the political spectrum, even though economics and sociology have long accommodated and encouraged empiricism. (p. 96)

What has passed for data in this sphere is little more than unverified physician self-reports—what I would term "Feels bad" surveys—of very questionable reliability (Black, 1990).

By contrast, in a rare study examining actual rather than self-reported behavior, researchers found no association between the malpractice experience of exposure of individual physicians and any increase in their use of prenatal resources or cesarean sections for the care of low-risk obstetrical patients. One explanation for this finding is that physicians exaggerate their reactions to liability anxiety, that is, they overreport how much this anxiety influences their practices (Baldwin, Hart, Lloyd, Fordyce, & Rosenblatt, 1995). Another study challenges the conventional wisdom (Localio, Lawthers, Bengtson, Hebert, Weaver, Brennan, et al., 1993), fueled by organized medicine's self-serving propaganda (Hale, 1994), that cesarean section rates have been driven wildly out of line by physicians' liability concerns (Entman, Glass, Hickson, Githens, Whetten-Goldstein, & Sloan, 1994, p. 1591). A different study, though, concludes that malpractice exposure influences slightly the use of electronic fetal monitoring (EFM), a major diagnostic tool (Tussing & Wojtowycz, 1997).

The most difficult impediment to getting a firm handle on the defensive medicine phenomenon is the difficulty of distinguishing, on one hand, practices resulting from the physician's legal fears from, on the other hand, medical care that would be provided in exactly the same way but for different reasons (U.S. General Accounting Office, 1995a, pp. 2, 10–13). According to Brennan (1991, p. 135), "Most physicians would probably have a hard time coming up with a list of procedures that are highly influenced by defensive medicine." Even assuming that we could accurately make this distinction as applied to particular patient care situations, drawing a bright line between "negative" and "positive" defensive medicine is (as we shall see later in this chapter) hardly a simple exercise (Hubbard, 1989, p. 313). From ethical, economic, and clinical perspectives, "We have no acceptable definition of inappropriate care" (Pauly, 1995, p. 70).

The issue of legal apprehensions as possible physician pretext is a vexing but vital one. These apprehensions and anxieties get blamed for a great deal of defensive medical practice. In formulating policy reactions to the defensive practice problem, it is imperative that we attempt to discern, first, whether physicians actually are practicing defensively and, second (assuming an affirmative answer to the first question), the real as opposed to claimed cause(s) of those defensive practices.

In the next section, I look at physician self-reports of defensive medicine. As we have already noted, though, these reports must be examined with caution. Several studies have produced findings that fly in the face of physician claims about their own conduct. Two investigations, for instance, found that, contrary to what family physicians often claim, malpractice premium costs were not associated with family physicians' likelihood of providing maternity care (Grumbach, Vranizan, Rennie, & Luft, 1997; Pathman & Tropman, 1995). The Office of Technology Assessment (U.S. Congress, 1994) estimated that less than 8 percent of diagnostic procedures is likely to be caused primarily by conscious concern and calculation about malpractice consequences.

Even assuming for the sake of argument that American physicians' self-reports about defensive medicine are true, apprehensions about adverse legal consequences may not be to blame, at least fully. In fact, defensive practices may be the complex product of an array of diverse forces that all push synergistically in the same direction (Black, 1990, p. 36; U.S. Department of Health and Human Services, 1987, p. 98). Put differently, defensive medical practices may represent physician conduct that would have occurred for other reasons even in the absence of sincere legal fears. As Putterman and Ben-Chetrit (1995), two rheumatologists, state:

> Testing habits that are difficult to erase, the simple availability of sophisticated technology . . . pressure from patients and their families, time constraints that limit the physician's willingness to contemplate data before ordering a test, the fear of missing a crucial diagnosis, and simple zeal for the attainment of diagnostic certainty are all inducements to test. (p. 1211)

This view accords with the experienced internist who informed me, "Medical practice would change little if all the lawyers in the world were sent to perdition right away."

One family physician told me that physicians order tests because "we are scared that the patient might be right about her problem." Several others confessed to being driven mainly by worry about being embarrassed by being shown to deviate from their medical peers; "No one wants to be out front in doing less." In terms of quality and ethics, this seems a form of "keeping *down* with the Joneses," where physicians perceive that they are more likely to be awarded peer respect for excessive intervention than for justifying the withholding of various tests and procedures. Physicians complain of never overcoming the "resident mentality of being grilled on morning report" for failing to turn up some arcane fact about the patient; excessive preoperative workups are often cited as an example of the manifestation of this mentality.

It is more comfortable for physicians to scapegoat the law than to admit the iatrogenic elements for which they ought to bear partial responsibility. The physician's uneasiness with uncertainty and sincere intellectual curiosity ("We must see the image and know") are legitimate concerns, for instance, but are they ethical when certainty is pursued at the patient's expense rather than for her benefit so that the physician's curiosity can be placated? Especially when physician actions are driven by personal philosophical views or the desire to avoid uncomfortable interpersonal situations, physicians may prefer to attribute those actions to a "neutral" explanation like the law; often it is easier to deal with moral conflicts by couching disagreements in morally neutral terms (Orentlicher, 1994, p. 1289). When physicians rely on the perceived threat of legal liability as a way to justify or rationalize actions based mainly on other motives, they might be viewed as hiding behind the law as a form of psychological, as well as legal, self-protection (McCrary, Swanson, Perkins, & Winslade, 1992, p. 373). It is also less arduous to dream of changing malpractice law (see Chapter 7) than to admit that significant alterations are needed in the fundamental ideology and organization of health care delivery.

As I have suggested elsewhere (Kapp, 1994):

> There certainly is a dispute about the extent to which the ordering of extra tests and procedures that are widely attributed to the physician's felt need to engage in defensive medicine are more accurately an artifact of the traditional fee-for-service payment system, in which the physician's compensation is directly related to the expenses the physician can induce the patient to incur. Similarly, are extra tests and procedures driven less by defensive medicine than by the prevalent technological imperative philosophy that more is always better and that, once invented and purchased, no machine should ever sit idle? (p. 71)

The depth of feeling on this point is illustrated in the statement by an official of the federal Department of Health and Human Services Inspector General's Office:

> If a doctor is running unsound tests, not for the beneficiary [patient] but for his or her own benefit, then the doctor should pay for it, not [the government's Medicare or Medicaid programs]. Health practitioners hold themselves out as experts and are highly paid for that expertise. They should be using their judgment to provide services as efficiently and cost-effectively as possible. (Patton, 1992)

An even stronger condemnation comes from a surgeon-turned-plaintiffs' attorney:

> As the AMA describes it, defensive medicine does not exist. It is a contradiction in terms. If tests are being performed that assist the doctor in determining a diagnosis or treatment, then they are not unnecessary. They are part of a good examination, the patient benefits from them, and they have nothing to do with protection against lawsuits.
>
> If doctors perform unnecessary tests, they are likely doing it for the money. Cases abound of physicians ordering patients to undergo tests and procedures that they don't need, then billing the patient or the insurance company for the additional cost. This practice is nothing new. It used to be called fraud; now the AMA calls it defensive medicine. (Wachsman, 1993, p. 164)

According to another medical gadfly:

> I do not think malpractice fears are relevant, although clearly physicians think they are, and I do not dispute their beliefs. But several lines of reasoning, of evidence, make one wonder how important a factor malpractice is. One is that a significant number of unnecessary cesarean sections are in women who never go into labor; they are automatically scheduled for repeat cesarean sections when their pregnancy is known. They are hardly at high risk; they should not be treated differently from women who have never had a cesarean section. Second, a study in California shows a significantly higher cesarean section rate in for-profit hospitals than in non-profit hospitals. The doctors in all those hospitals pay the same malpractice premiums. (Wolfe, 1991, p. 459)

At the same time, though, one study indicated that equalizing payments for cesarean and vaginal deliveries had little effect on cesarean rates (Keeler & Fok, 1996), thereby supporting the idea that malpractice fears do strongly drive behavior in this area.

The technological imperative (the "romance of technology") to treat the patient as a source of data that should be collected for its own sake is ingrained in the process of medical education from the first lecture (although the advent of managed care may be changing this—see Chapter 6). Students and residents are taught early and repeatedly to err on the side of more, that not having a piece of data will require an explanation to the medical mentor (regardless of legal considerations), but one will never have to justify collecting too much data (Krieger, 1996). This approach fits squarely with the tradition of medical perfectionism described in the previous chapter. Thus does ritual (e.g., in the ordering of laboratory tests) often trump scientific reasoning.

A recent interesting study examined residents' compliance with consensus ethics guidelines of the American College of Physicians. Resident respondents reported a variety of explanations for their frequent ethical lapses, most notably sleep deprivation and overwork, that did not involve legal apprehensions (Green, Mitchell, Stocking, Cassel, & Siegler, 1996). A study in which British physicians blamed their ordering of diagnostic tests of questionable clinical value on legal motivations surmises, "Litigation may not be the only causal factor for the observed changes in practice" (Ennis, Clark, & Grudzinskas, 1991, p. 616); other possible factors noted were training, work environment, peer esteem, and the physical stress or fatigue of the physician. Indeed, the fact that several other countries with different (i.e., presumably less tense) liability climates have higher cesarean section rates than the United States hints at explanations other than defensive medicine (Martensen, 1994).

To the extent that defensive medicine is used by physicians as a pretext to justify conduct that is mainly otherwise determined, the rationalization process may be largely unconscious. As one physician noted to me, "We are all good at making our own alibis." Elsewhere (Kapp, 1993), I have suggested as a way to address this issue a legal requirement that physicians explicitly include a statement of their legal anxiety motivations and considerations as part of the information that they share with the patient in obtaining informed consent to any medical test, procedure, or other intervention. In other words, I propose that, where the physician suggests a particular intervention to a patient primarily because the physician fears potential liability if the intervention is not initiated (that is, making a recommendation for defensive medicine purposes), and the same intervention would not be recommended in a litigation-free world, this fact should be imparted to the patient. Then, that patient can take the physician's motivation into account in making an informed, voluntary, competent choice about whether or not to undergo the intervention.

"COVERING OUR REARS": HOW PHYSICIANS DESCRIBE DEFENSIVE MEDICINE

The previous section has pointed out some of the evidentiary and analytical limitations of relying too heavily on physicians' own self-reports about the negative implications of defensive medicine. These limitations notwithstanding, because perception is in many respects more important than reality, we must examine—seriously but with care—how physicians think that legal anxieties affect their practices. This thinking breaks defensive behavior down into several categories: overtesting, overtreatment, impaired information exchange with patients (specifically in the contexts of suboptimal informed consent and the hiding of medical errors), general harm to the physician-patient relationship, restricted access either for certain patients or to certain types of care, and unnecessary deficiencies in medical education, research, and innovation.

Overtesting

Physicians say that the threat of malpractice lawsuits causes them to order diagnostic tests they might otherwise consider unnecessary (American College of Physicians, 1995, p. 467; Lawthers, Localio, Laird, Lipsitz, Hebert, & Brennan, 1992; Weisman, Morlock, Teitelbaum, Klassen, & Celentano, 1989; Peters, Nord, & Woodson, 1986, p. 616), in search of the "unambiguous certainty" that modern technology promises (Denny, 1994). This practice seems especially ironic, because the amount of uncertainty about which diagnostic tests actually provide useful information is itself still relatively high (Reid, Lachs, & Feinstein, 1995). Some physicians realize that the additional data derived from excessive testing probably will be of marginal or no benefit to the patient's care, but they believe that they (physicians) need the tests to bolster the documentation through which plaintiffs' attorneys may someday forage (U.S. Congress, 1994, p. 32); why else would physicians order tests redundantly (at the same time) rather than sequentially? In a world in which a premium is continually placed on quantification and illusory objectivity, physicians feel that the legal system and patient expectations have combined to devalue clinical judgment and the art of medicine.

Some ritualistic diagnostic testing, though not helpful, is not tangibly harmful either, such as a surgeon giving one last listen to the patient's heart prior to surgery even though the patient has been thoroughly worked up preoperatively and cleared by a primary care physician, or obtaining one last chest X ray before surgery even though others have been taken recently. Most scattershot diagnostic tests, however, are not benign. They inflict potential harm on the patient, besides the direct financial expense, in the forms of: risk of physical or emotional (Melendez & McCrank, 1993) morbidity or mortality from the test itself; pain, discomfort, and inconvenience; dangers involved in traveling to and from the test; emotional turmoil (for the family, too) waiting for the test to be done, and then for the results to be received, interpreted, and conveyed by the physician back to the patient; and the chance to do it all again if the first set of tests yields a false positive (DeAngelis, 1987). A VQ Scan for a postoperative patient with a very small chance of pulmonary embolism is cited by many physicians as a classic example of defensively driven excessive testing. Sometimes, further tests are needed to resolve discrepancies between earlier tests, and the dance can continue indefinitely. As attorney / tort system critic Peter Huber (1991, p. 90) assesses the circumstances, "Far from accelerating the shift to better medicine, litigation has frozen in place an unhelpful techno-fix and contributed to the dis-education of medical practitioners."

Physicians' perceived overtesting behavior for legally defensive reasons is associated with another widespread physician belief, namely, that anxiety about litigation and liability has sorely wounded the spirit of collegiality that used to commonly characterize the relationship among physicians. Today, it is argued, physicians experience and engage in less collegiality among and toward their peers because so much of their behavior is driven by a felt need to document a defensible record that would allow one physician to share potential risks with, or even better shift potential risks to, other physicians in the event of a bad patient outcome. Primary care physicians may overuse specialty and subspecialty consultations for this purpose, seeking confirmation for the record rather than real guidance in patient care. For the same perceived risk management reason, the consultant(s) may return reports to the referring physician that are unnecessarily ambiguous and hedging, leaving the primary caregiver no choice but to step up the diagnostic assault a few notches. Having posed the question, the primary care physician would be petrified to ignore the proffered response. Counterproductive defensive behavior also takes place when a consultant physician tries to protect himself by disparaging the work of a colleague who has treated that patient previously, and the patient is thereby provoked into suing one or both physicians because of an adverse event (Beckman, Markakis, Suchman, & Frankel, 1994).

Overtreatment

Tests have sequelae. The most negative aspect of defensive diagnostic testing is that it often leads to defensive treatment. An increase in downstream procedures has been closely tracked to the substantial increase in diagnostic testing in this country (Verrilli & Welch, 1996). For example, a study supported by the federal Agency for Health Care Policy and Research found that patients who undergo coronary stress testing (treadmill tests) are more likely to undergo subsequent coronary angiography and, similarly, patients who have angiography are more likely to undergo a revascularization procedure such as angioplasty or coronary artery bypass graft (CABG) surgery. According to that study's authors, this association between testing and subsequent therapeutic procedures reflects underlying uncertainties about when to test for and treat ischemic heart disease (Wennberg, Kellett, Dickens, Malenka, Keilson, & Keller, 1996).

Treatment interventions—procedures and/or drugs—initiated more for the physician's perceived legal benefit than for the patient's therapeutic benefit are unnecessarily risky and, therefore, bad practice (Ennis, Clark, & Grudzinskas, 1991). As such, unduly risky treatments initiated without a proper scientific rationale serve to expand rather than limit the physician's potential legal exposure in the event of a proximately-caused injury to the patient, but most physicians somehow fail to understand this part of the risk equation.

Impaired Communications—The Perversion of Informed Consent

One indisputable product of the modern legal climate is an enhanced emphasis on the autonomy or self-determination of the patient, as effectuated through the legal doctrine of informed consent. Most physicians are deeply ambivalent about the ethical ramifications of this legally enforced emphasis. Though many acknowledge, happily or begrudgingly, its positive effects, physicians in large measure are critical of ways in which they believe the legal aspects of informed consent impair rather than enhance the ethical content of their patient interactions.

These criticisms stem primarily from a perverse misinterpretation of the informed consent doctrine (Meisel & Kuczewski, 1996; Rosoff, 1994) and fall into two categories. There is a pervasive belief that the law requires (a) that patients be tortured with unnecessary and inappropriate information and (b) that the physician slavishly provide whatever unnecessary and inappropriate interventions the patient may demand.

Many physicians feel that their legal vulnerabilities compel them to tell (many use the phrase "dump on") their patients (and often the families, with or without the patient's authentic blessing [Kaufman, 1993, p. 308]) too many facts about their conditions, "often more than they need to know" (Tenery, 1995). This is not a new complaint (Kaplan, Greenwald, & Rogers, 1977), but it has grown in strength over the years. Ethically, physicians question whether "the gains in patient autonomy and improved outcomes produced by the dialogue are worth the additional time, money, and needless patient anxiety and confusion that informed consent may entail" (Schuck, 1994, p. 904). There is a common sentiment that "conscientiously followed, our present policy of full disclosure too often results in a confusing and bewildering information overload, or produces states of fear, anxiety, or depression that impede rational thought and can impede recovery" (Philips, 1994). Put by one psychiatrist in a more self-interested vein, "For three decades, the law has pretended that the doctrine [of informed consent] assists patient care. However, this is fiction; the doctrine has sorely burdened physicians" (Piper, 1994, p. 311).

Much of this burden—as well as that imposed on patients—may be attributed to significant misunderstandings about the substance of informed consent law. For instance, some physicians now believe that they are obligated to virtually coerce patients to physically return to the medical office in order to be given negative test results, because telephone contact will not look as impressive in the record if something goes wrong later. Pediatrician/attorney Ellen Wright Clayton (1995, p. S14-S15) suggests a truly perverse example: physicians who fear they will not be able to prove legally valid informed refusal for genetic testing feeling that they must therefore perform available tests even when their patients do not want them.

In cases of terminal illness, "recent research indicates that total frankness about prognosis is generally viewed by physicians as neither appropriate nor therapeutic" (Kaufman, 1993, p. 310). Nonetheless, physicians feel the need to paint the bleakest picture ("hanging crepe") (Siegler, 1975) to the patient and/or family in order to avoid the sort of later surprise and disappointment that—physicians perceive—could fuel a trip to the lawyer's office.

In circumstances where physicians take offense at what they have convinced themselves are unreasonable legal shackles binding them, they usually have the practical power to act in ways that undermine and defeat the law's intent. Certainly, this dynamic occurs frequently in the context of informed consent, with physicians complying with the formal letter of the law in terms of straight information disclosure but consciously and effectively sabotaging the spirit of patient autonomy that animates informed consent legislation and judicial precedent (Katz, 1992). Legal scholar A. J. Rosoff (1994) has accurately described what happens:

> Formal compliance with the law's requirements—a signed consent form, a completed check list of disclosure items, and so forth—is objectively verifiable; it yields hard evidence that what is required was in fact done. Contrast this with a difficult-to-document ongoing process of respectful, open, two-way communication. It is no wonder that people concerned with protecting themselves from litigation will focus on the more readily documentable aspects. In theory, it need not be an either-or situation. There is no reason, in concept, why full and open communication is inconsistent with documenting the disclosure of specific data; but, in a busy world where time is at a premium, the concrete often does displace the abstract. Thus, once the forms are signed and entered into a patient's record, it is all too easy to feel that the goal of informed consent has been achieved. It has not. (p. 316)

The proof of the pudding is in the eating. As a 1996 study found, legislation in several jurisdictions mandating physicians to disclose options for the treatment of breast cancer (obviously intended to promote patient self-determination) had only a slight and transient effect on the rate of use of breast-conserving surgery (Nattinger, Hoffmann, Shapiro, Gottlieb, & Goodwin, 1996). The conclusion logically drawn from this result is that even if other alternatives are formally recited, the physician's recommendation is the course of treatment that usually ends up being pursued; as physicians tell me constantly, "We can talk our patients into anything."

But physicians' complaints about the long arm of the law are nothing if not radically inconsistent. Despite their acknowledged ability to undermine the spirit of informed consent law in practice, many physicians simultaneously insist that legal requirements are ethically counterproductive because they often lead to bad patient/family decisions that the physician is required to implement under penalty of malpractice litigation and liability. Physicians frequently report frustration at feeling legally compelled to "cave in" to unreasonable, unrealistic patient/family demands for inappropriate treatments. It is a hassle to say no to demands driven by the patient's hopes and fears, even though most physicians understand that good communication generally can "cover the bases" and ultimately convince most patients of the wisdom of holding back on various inappropriate tests and procedures (Kasper, Mulley, & Wennberg, 1992; Barry, Mulley, Fowler, & Wennberg, 1988). When the patient pushes or acts stubbornly, the path of least resistance in every respect—financial incentives, the physician's time and energy, and perceived risk management needs—is to be accommodating, that is, to "just do it": every respect, that is, except the ethical.

Physician Robert Kane (1995) articulates it clearly:

> Especially in a market where patients can choose virtually any physician, doctors are under some compulsion to provide patients with the services they desire. Moreover, this demand is exacerbated by an active news media that promulgates each new discovery, sometimes suggesting that early results promise great cures. Physicians may in fact have to expend considerable effort to dissuade patients from a particular treatment because it is not in their best interests. Such activity is many things but lucrative. Not only is a physician's time spent talking poorly rewarded, compared to the performance of a procedure, but also, if the end result is patient frustration at not receiving the desired service, then the effort is doubly uncompensated. (p. 63)

Ordering prostate specific antigen (PSA) tests for men without specific clinical indications is an example of perceived overuse and misuse of diagnostic testing driven by fear of liability despite the absence of convincing scientific evidence supporting use of the test. Physicians suggest that they go along with their patients' excessive expectations regarding diagnostic tests because "safely not ordering the PSA test would entail serious discussion time" with the patient to explain why the test was not indicated. The perceived safest, and certainly the easiest, thing to do "in terms of covering your fanny" is simply to avoid that conversation and order the test.

Another example comes from the realm of ophthalmology. Some patients insist on surgery to remove benign tumors that are incidentally discovered through imaging that has been ordered for a completely different reason, where the tumor is harmless and produces no symptoms (Bullock & Haik, 1995; Yohai, Bullock, & Margolis, 1993). Going along with excessive use of technology in these cases is considered ethically objectionable when it creates unnecessary risks (let alone expense) for the patient. In the same vein, a leader in the modern history of obstetrics in the United States confided not long ago, "I think to some extent obstetricians have abrogated their responsibility to the patient by simply saying, 'This is her choice'" about such matters as the need for an episiotomy (Kaufman, 1993, p. 205).

Impaired Communications—Hiding Medical Errors

Errors have always been a part of medical practice (Bosk, 1979). Physicians instinctively and universally believe that the current tort system punishes medical errors. Consequently, physicians maintain, they are too intimidated by fear of adverse legal repercussions to admit their mistakes; instead, the legal incentives are perceived as pushing physicians strongly in the direction of covering up errors (Ending the blame game, 1996; Levy, 1995; Marks, 1995; Leape, 1994; Senders, 1994, p. 171).

> Those who are associated with errors are the most likely people to be able to provide information about what contributes to the errors. There is an impediment to their providing information, however, which is fear of malpractice litigation. Most medical care providers in the United States will not provide error-related information because to do so might be construed as admitting responsibility for any error under consideration. This could lead to litigation. (Bogner, 1994, p. 379)

Renowned Harvard surgeon Francis D. Moore (1995, p. 91) has written about mortality and morbidity (M & M) conferences as essential to continuing medical education and correcting errors. He laments, however, the fact that physicians now feel that honestly discussing with their colleagues things that have gone wrong in patient care puts them at intolerable risk legally.

Hiding or rationalizing, rather than acknowledging, medical errors is ethically harmful for at least three kinds of reasons. First, it interferes with the desirable process of turning errors into educational "treasures" (Blumenthal, 1994) from which both erring physicians and their colleagues might learn much and grow professionally. Second, it hurts patients by depriving them and their physicians of information that could potentially be valuable in correcting errors and otherwise improving treatment of present and future patients (Fetters, 1995). This offends the principles of beneficence and nonmaleficence (Snyder & Brennan, 1996). Families may also be cheated; for instance, fear of uncovering errors that might lead to litigation probably helps account for a decrease in the number of autopsies performed today, thereby diminishing many opportunities to learn, to comfort families with explanations of the patient's death, and to alert families to discovered genetic risks. Finally, purposeful deception undercuts and attacks the essential fabric of the fiduciary or trust nature of the physician-patient relationship by directly violating the ethical principle of fidelity or truthfulness (Ritchie & Davies, 1995).

Like many of the legal perceptions held by physicians about malpractice exposure, the notion that defensively covering up medical errors must be good risk management is a highly questionable one. Ironically, that strategy probably is counterproductive (Ritchie & Davies, 1994). There is evidence that most patients want their physicians to admit errors to them, and that complying with that patient preference may reduce rather than multiply the physician's risk of punitive actions (Witman, Park, & Hardin, 1996).

Damaging the Physician-Patient Relationship

Defensive medicine, according to physicians, has negative ramifications for the health of the physician-patient relationship in many ways, some of which have been discussed already. It is claimed that some of the traditional trust and communication have been superseded by physicians' felt need to constantly look over their shoulders for the patient's attorney from the time a relationship is first initiated (Mc-Quade, 1991). An adversary legal climate makes physicians unenthusiastic about practicing medicine and helping patients (Berczeller, 1994, pp. 210–211; Fruchter, 1993, p. 488). One physician, in describing his changed life after defending against a malpractice claim, quotes a patient complaining to the office nurse, "I can't stand this new [physician]. He spends all his time scribbling instead of talking to me" (Anderson, 1996, p. 16).

In his classic study of medical error, sociologist Charles Bosk (1979, p. 98) reflected on the physician's loss of personal charisma and the evolution of a more formally contractual relationship. This change—a distancing of the physician from the patient—is regrettable for those who believe that physician behavior would be driven ordinarily by an embrace of the physician's fiduciary duties, although it likely would be endorsed by critics who see physicians as being unduly influenced by self-interest.

Impaired Access to Medical Care

The tort system is based on the rationale that improper conduct will be deterred by fear of punishment. One problem, though, is that deterrence may go awry. "Overdeterrence may result in . . . the unavailability of useful goods or services" (Shuman, 1993a, p. 167). Because of defensive medicine, appropriate access may be improperly limited either for particular individuals or regarding particular kinds of potentially useful treatments (Brown, 1996; Tancredi & Barondess, 1978). In either case, the ethical principle of social or distributive justice may be sorely compromised.

Many physicians claim that they shy away from serving certain categories of patients because they "can smell a lawsuit down the road." In those situations, risk avoidance is a value that trumps social obligation (Weisman, Morlock, Teitelbaum, Klassen, & Celentano, 1989; Perry & Lehrman, 1987; Peters, Nord, & Woodson, 1986, p. 616; Charles, Wilbert, & Franke, 1985, p. 440). Some physicians, for example, refuse to treat attorneys or their families (Macklin, 1993, p. 14). Many psychiatrists try to avoid violent and suicidal patients for legally defensive reasons. A county health commissioner told me that private physicians frequently send insured pediatric patients, for whom they otherwise provide a full range of services, to the public health department for their pertussis vaccinations because the private physicians fear litigation stemming from rare but serious adverse reactions. Because this entails a separate trip for parent and child, some children go unvaccinated as a result.

In response to discrimination against the poor supposedly induced by defensive medicine, the Federally Supported Health Centers Assistance Act of 1995, Public Law 104-73, effectively takes patients in community health centers out of the conventional tort system. Employees, contractors, and other entities associated with such centers are deemed by the Act to be employees of the Public Health Service, thereby bringing them under the Federal Tort Claims Act, which limits non-economic damages and makes the government the sole defendant in the event of a suit.

The poor may be disadvantaged in another way. If fear of litigation really does bring about excessive medical testing and treatment, health care costs are driven up unnecessarily. More expensive care thus becomes even less accessible to individuals who lack adequate health insurance or deep enough financial pockets (Weiler, Hiatt, Newhouse, Johnson, Brennan, & Leape, 1993, p. 134).

Unfortunately, many physicians do not equate good medical practice with effective risk management. "In particular, physicians may forego certain indicated procedures because of the risk of a lawsuit" (Harris, 1987, p. 2802). As a consequence, patients may have access to beneficial medical services impeded because large numbers of physicians are too legally apprehensive to provide those services. One well-known example involves physicians restricting their delivery of obstetrical services purportedly as a function of risk management, thereby creating an access crisis for some patients, particularly those in rural areas (Lewis-Idema, 1989, p. 78).

Other examples include: drug and device manufacturers pulling products that benefit large numbers of people from the marketplace or failing to develop them in the first place because of a very small risk of very expensive injury to a few possible plaintiffs (even in the absence of credible proof linking those injuries to the drug or product involved) (Angell, 1996); physicians being too afraid to consider "alternative" treatments even at the patient's request (Goodenough & Park, 1996); physicians failing to stop and render aid in emergency situations (Dillard, 1995), despite the existence of Good Samaritan statutes in every jurisdiction that immunize physicians against liability and the fact that no physician in the United States has ever been successfully sued for rendering emergency aid as a Good Samaritan; and fear of liability deterring retired physicians from volunteering their time and thus improving patient access to medical care (Manuel, 1994).

Regulations may also have a chilling effect on patients' access to beneficial services. This is illustrated by the decrease in availability of office cultures for group A streptococci following implementation of the Clinical Laboratory Improvement Amendments (CLIA) of 1988 (Schwartz, Fries, Fitzgibbon, & Lipman, 1994).

Interestingly, these defensive practices are not limited to physicians who must cope with the American tort system. Some Canadian physicians, for instance, stopped taking on new prenatal patients in the summer of 1996 after their government reduced its subsidies for their malpractice insurance costs (Greenberg, 1996).

Medical Education, Research, and Innovation

Medical educators claim that the constant awareness of lawsuit risk is a shadow hanging over the process of educating students and residents (Challoner, Kilpatrick, Dockery, & Dwyer, 1988). The process of medical research may also be skewed in a negative direction, as occurs for example when investigators exclude women of childbearing age from participation in research protocols from which they might benefit, based on visions of deformed fetuses making plaintiffs' attorneys rich.

Fear of legal consequences often inspires—foolishly, in many situations—overly conservative, dogmatically rigid physician behavior, under the theory that what has always been done before is more legally prophylactic (even when there is no scientific evidence of the standard approach's effectiveness or safety) than acting creatively or innovatively. "[R]isky choices with a potential for better outcomes are rejected in favor of options that are believed to be fail-safe, not in the sense that they are necessarily best for the patient involved, but best in the sense that the person making the decision is safe from legal recourse even if things turn out badly" (Moray, 1994, p. 85). Legal anxieties push individual physicians to follow the crowd; because no one wants to play Lone Ranger with a lucrative career, medical practices frequently get adopted, taught, and perpetuated based on group enthusiasm and momentum instead of supportive evidence (Konner, 1993, pp. 127–128).

TIME-OUT AT THE PHYSICIANS' PITY PARTY: RATIONALES FOR THE TORT SYSTEM

The medical profession, and many other participants and observers, are correct that the present system for resolving legal claims of medical malpractice leaves much to be desired. Although I think there is much misunderstanding of tort law, its operation, and its implications by practicing physicians, for the most part I agree with them that the legal *status quo* carries great potential for inducing suboptimal, even at times unethical, behavior in the realm of patient care. As explained by Daniel Shuman (1993a, p. 154), the threat of "punishment has short term desirable effects, but also long term undesirable effects including anxiety and timidity. The anxiety expressed by physicians over medical malpractice is characteristic of what behaviorists regard as the consequences of a system that relies on punishment." Additionally,

> Cognitive psychology reveals that human decisionmaking is systematically flawed, and that faulty information processing is the norm. Thus, the risk of tort sanctions is not likely to induce safer behavior in appropriate cases. Rather, cognitive psychology reveals that we are likely to overestimate tort risks and avoid desirable activity. (Shuman, 1993a, p. 166)

Warts and all, though, the tort system has evolved over history to serve specific purposes—even if, in modern practice, evidence regarding whether it actually serves those purposes very effectively and efficiently is quite inconclusive (Shuman, 1994; 1993b; 1992, pp. 410–411). One purpose is to improve the quality of patient care by deterring substandard, unsafe medical practices (Brennan & Berwick, 1996, p. 71; Wachsman, 1993, pp. 169–170). To the extent that the physician response to a perceived threat of lawsuits acts to forestall or prevent some avoidable patient injuries, defensive medicine may be interpreted positively (U.S. General Accounting Office, 1995b; Weiler, Hiatt, Newhouse, Johnson, Brennan, & Leape, 1993, p. 133). J. M. McGreevy (1994), a medical professor, advises fledgling physicians:

If you are worried that malpractice is going to interfere with your enjoyment of a medical career, forget it. In my opinion, malpractice concerns will force you to practice with more precision and more intelligence. You will be ready to justify all of your actions, but this is just the way you should want it to be. If you don't want it that way, then you should consider another career. (p. 32)

As one physician confided to me privately, asking himself, "How would this play to a jury?" has sharpened his thinking markedly.

Another purpose of the tort system is to provide a means of financial compensation to patients who are iatrogenically injured through no fault of their own. This is a widely agreed-on social imperative in a country without a well-developed first-party social insurance system. The problem in practice lies with trying to fulfill a broad societal responsibility by placing it on the backs of individual tort defendants in the context of specific civil judgments.

In addition, the law can serve society as a sort of "moral tutor," especially in civil rights arenas (Schneider, 1996, p. 37). Surely, malpractice law has fulfilled this role in improving health care providers' respect for the fundamental moral value of patient and family autonomy (Kaufman, 1993, p. 255). To the extent that the older paternalistic approach has been displaced by patients and families truly participating in medical decisions affecting their own lives today, much of the credit belongs to the courts and legislatures.

Although physicians complain bitterly about the civil justice environment, most admit to themselves—even though not often publicly—that the malpractice system is not entirely evil incarnate. Some benefits to patients and society have been stimulated. The key, when we examine public policy alternatives (see Chapter 7), is to suggest bold strategies for throwing out the bathwater trying to mitigate negative behavioral effects of physicians' malpractice apprehensions without at the same time throwing out the baby (the salutary clinical and ethical effects on patient care associated with our tort system).

CONCLUSION

When legal anxieties drive physicians to make practice changes that improve the quality and ethics of medical care delivery, a salutary public policy purpose is served. For the most part, however, this is not the case. As a general proposition, physicians LaPuma and Schiedermayer (1989) are correct when they admonish:

Malpractice prevention is an ethical dilemma; perceived legal obligations can distort a physician's clinical judgment. Performing procedures [or other defensive practices] for legal reasons is unethical and does not necessarily prevent malpractice suits. Physicians must resist these pressures. (p. 414)

NOTE

1. These sentiments also apply to perceived regulatory intrusions, such as federal provisions criminalizing Medicare/Medicaid fraud and abuse. The head of the Association of American Physicians and Surgeons, a libertarian fringe of the medical profession, has written (Orient, 1994): "One cardiac surgeon stated that he would no longer use stents to keep coronary arteries open in Medicare patients. He is not willing to risk his career. Instead he will perform open-heart surgery on these patients, a much more invasive procedure."

REFERENCES

American College of Physicians (1995). Beyond MICRA: New ideas for liability reform. *Annals of Internal Medicine, 122*, 466–473.

Anderson, E. (1996, March 4). Physician won malpractice case, but still lost a lot. *American Medical News, 39*, 15–16.

Angell, M. (1996). Evaluating the health risks of breast implants: The interplay of medical science, the law, and public opinion. *New England Journal of Medicine, 334*, 1513–1518.

Baldwin, L.-M., Hart, G., Lloyd, M., Fordyce, M., & Rosenblatt, R.A. (1995). Defensive medicine and obstetrics. *Journal of the American Medical Association, 274*, 1606–1610.

Barry, M. J., Mulley, A. G. J., Fowler, F. J., & Wennberg, J. W. (1988). Watchful waiting vs. immediate transurethral resection for symptomatic prostatism: The importance of patients' preferences. *Journal of the American Medical Association, 259*, 3010–3017.

Beckman, H. B., Markakis, K. M., Suchman, A. L., & Frankel, R. M. (1994). The doctor-patient relationship and malpractice: Lessons from plaintiff depositions. *Archives of Internal Medicine, 154*, 1365–1370.

Berczeller, P. H. (1994). *Doctors and patients: What we feel about you.* New York: Macmillan Publishing Company.

Black, N. (1990). Medical litigation and the quality of care. *Lancet, 335*, 35–37.

Blumenthal, D. (1994). Making medical errors into "medical treasures." *Journal of the American Medical Association, 272*, 1867–1868.

Bogner, M. S. (1994). Human error in medicine: A frontier for change. In M. S. Bogner (Ed.), *Human Error in Medicine* (pp. 373–383). Hillsdale, NJ: Lawrence Erlbaum Associates.

Bosk, C. L. (1979). *Forgive and remember: Managing medical failure.* Chicago: University of Chicago Press.

Brennan, T. A. (1995). Book review of *Suing for malpractice,* by F. Sloan, P. B. Githens, E. W. Clayton, G. B. Hickson, D. A. Gentile, & D. F. Partlett. *Journal of Law, Medicine & Ethics, 23*, 96–100.

Brennan, T. A. (1991). *Just doctoring: Medical ethics in the liberal state.* Berkeley: University of California Press.

Brennan, T. A., & Berwick, D. M. (1996). *New rules: Regulation, markets, and the quality of American health care.* San Francisco: Jossey-Bass Publishers.

Brown, J. L. (1996). Statutory immunity for volunteer physicians: A vehicle for reaafirmation of the doctor's beneficent duties—absent the rights talk. *Widener Law Symposium Journal, 1,* 425–463.

Bullock, J. D., & Haik, H. M., Jr. (1995). Incidental orbital cavernous hemangiomas. *Orbit, 14,* 87–91.

Challoner, D. R., Kilpatrick, K. E., Dockery, J. L., & Dwyer, J. W. (1988). Effects of the liability climate on the academic health center. *New England Journal of Medicine, 319,* 1603–1605.

Charles, S. C., Wilbert, J. R., & Franke, K. J. (1985). Sued and nonsued physicians' self-reported reactions to malpractice litigation. *American Journal of Psychiatry, 142,* 437–440.

Clayton, E. W. (1995, May–June). The dispersion of genetic technologies and the law. *Hastings Center Report, 25,* S13–S15.

DeAngelis, C. (1987). Medical malpractice litigation: Does it augment or impede quality care? *Journal of Pediatrics, 110,* 878–880.

Denny, W. F. (1994, May–June). Letter, the sorcerer's lawyer. *Hastings Center Report, 24,* 50.

Dillard, J. N. (1995, June 12). *Newsweek,* 12.

Ending the blame game. [Editorial]. (1996, November 18). *American Medical News, 39,* p. 17.

Ennis, M., Clark, A., & Grudzinskas, J. G. (1991). Change in obstetric practice in response to fear of litigation in the British Isles. *Lancet, 338,* 616–618.

Entman, S. S., Glass, C. A., Hickson, G. B., Githens, P. B., Whetten-Goldstein, K., & Sloan, F. A. (1994). The relationship between malpractice claims history and subsequent obstetrical care. *Journal of the American Medical Association, 272,* 1588–1591.

Evans, J. G. (1996). Health care for older people: A look across a frontier. *Journal of the American Medical Association, 275,* 1449–1450.

Fetters, M. D. (1995). Error in medicine [Letter]. *Journal of the American Medical Association, 274,* 458.

Fruchter, J. (1993). Doctors on trial: A comparison of American and Jewish legal approaches to medical malpractice. *American Journal of Law & Medicine, 19,* 453–495.

Goodenough, U., & Park, R. L. (1996, November 22). Magic versus medicine: What future doctors need to know about alternative treatments. *Chronicle of Higher Education,* p. B6.

Green, M. J., Mitchell, G., Stocking, C. B., Cassel, C. K., & Siegler, M. (1996). Do actions reported by physicians in training conflict with consensus guidelines on ethics? *Archives of Internal Medicine, 156,* 298–304.

Greenberg, L. M. (1996, November 11). Ontario doctors start slowdown over proposal. *Wall Street Journal,* p. B6.

Greene, H. L., Goldberg, R. J., Beattie, H., Russo, A. R., Ellison, R. C., & Dalen, J. E. (1989). Physician attitudes toward cost containment: The missing piece of the puzzle. *Archives of Internal Medicine, 149,* 1966–1968.

Grumbach, K., Vranizan, K., Rennie, D., & Luft, H. S. (1997). Charges for obstetric liability insurance and discontinuation of obstetric practice in New York. *Journal of Family Practice, 44,* 61–70.

Hale, R. W. (1994). Reducing the rate of cesarean deliveries: An obtainable but elusive goal. *Journal of the American Medical Association, 272,* 558–559.

Hall, M. A. (1991). The defensive effect of medical practice policies in malpractice litigation. *Law & Contemporary Problems, 54,* 119–145.

Harris, J. E. (1987). Defensive medicine: It costs, but does it work? *Journal of the American Medical Association, 257,* 2801–2802.

Hershey, N. (1972). The defensive practice of medicine: Myth or reality? *Milbank Memorial Quarterly, 50,* 69–97.

Hubbard, F. P. (1989). The physicians' point of view concerning medical malpractice: A sociological perspective on the symbolic importance of "tort reform." *Georgia Law Review, 23,* 295–358.

Huber, P. W. (1991). *Galileo's revenge: Junk science in the courtroom.* New York: Basic Books.

Jacobs, M. A. (1995, September 8). Lawyers and clients: Overbilling is widely known at major firms. *Wall Street Journal,* p. B5.

Kane, R. L. (1995). Creating practice guidelines: The dangers of over-reliance on expert judgment. *Journal of Law, Medicine & Ethics, 23,* 62–64.

Kaplan, S., Greenwald, R., & Rogers, A. (1977). Neglected aspects of informed consent. *New England Journal of Medicine, 296,* 1127.

Kapp, M. B. (1994). Defensive medicine in geriatric practice. In F. Homburger (Ed.), *The rational use of advanced medical technology with the elderly* (pp. 67–74). New York: Springer Publishing Company.

Kapp, M. B. (1993, Spring). Informed consent to defensive medicine: Letting the patient decide. *The Pharos, 56,* 12–14.

Kasper, J. F., Mulley, A. G., & Wennberg, J. E. (1992). Developing shared decision-making programs to improve the quality of health care. *Quality Review Bulletin, 18,* 183–190.

Katz, J. (1992). Duty and caring in the age of informed consent and medical science: Unlocking Peabody's secret. *Humane Medicine, 8,* 187–197.

Kaufman, S. R. (1993). *The healer's tale: Transforming medicine and culture.* Madison, WI: University of Wisconsin Press.

Keeler, E. B., & Fok, T. (1996). Equalizing physician fees had little effect on cesarean rates. *Medical Care Research and Review, 53,* 465–471.

Konner, M. (1993). *Medicine at the crossroads: The crisis in health care.* New York: Pantheon Books.

Krieger, L. M. (1996). Reforming house staff's practice of defensive medicine. *Journal of the American Medical Association, 275,* 662.

LaPuma, J., and Schiedermayer, D. L. (1989). Outpatient clinical ethics. *Journal of General Internal Medicine, 4,* 413–420.

Lawthers, A. G., Localio, A. R., Laird, N. M., Lipsitz, S., Hebert, L., & Brennan, T. A. (1992). Physicians' perceptions of the risk of being sued. *Journal of Health Politics, Policy and Law, 17,* 463–482.

Leape, L. L. (1994). Error in medicine. *Journal of the American Medical Association, 272,* 1851–1857.

Levy, R. (1995, Fall). Code blue. *Harvard Public Health Review, 7,* 36–41.

Lewis-Idema, D. (1989). Medical professional liability and access to obstetrical care: Is there a crisis? In V. Rostow & R. J. Bulger (Eds.), *Medical professional liability and the delivery of obstetrical care.* Washington, DC: National Academy Press.

Localio, A. R., Lawthers, A. G., Bengtson, J. M., Hebert, L. E., Weaver, S. L., Brennan, T. A., et al. (1993). Relationship between malpractice claims and cesarean delivery. *Journal of the American Medical Association, 269,* 366–373.

Macklin, R. (1993). *Enemies of patients.* New York: Oxford University Press.

Manuel, B. (1994, October 21). No good deed goes unpunished. *Wall Street Journal,* p. A10.

Marks, L. D. (1995). Admitting mistakes [Letter]. *Annals of Emergency Medicine, 26,* 758.

Martensen, R. L. (1994). For deliberate election: Cesarean sections in the 1890s. *Journal of the American Medical Association, 271,* 1557.

McCrary, S. V., Swanson, J. W., Perkins, H. S., & Winslade, W. J. (1992). Treatment decisions for terminally ill patients: Physicians' legal defensiveness and knowledge of medical law. *Law, Medicine & Health Care, 20,* 364–376.

McGreevy, J. M. (1994, Winter). Advice to a college student considering medicine as a career. *The Pharos, 57,* 32–34.

McQuade, J. S. (1991). The medical malpractice crisis—reflections on the alleged causes and proposed cures. *Journal of the Royal Society of Medicine, 84,* 408–411.

Meisel, A., & Kuczewski, M. (1996). Legal and ethical myths about informed consent. *Archives of Internal Medicine, 156,* 2521–2526.

Melendez, J. C., & McCrank, E. (1993). Anxiety-related reactions associated with magnetic resonance imaging examinations. *Journal of the American Medical Association, 270,* 745–747.

Milgrom, P., Whitney, C., Conrad, D., Fiset, L., & O'Hara, D. (1995). Tort reform and malpractice liability insurance. *Medical Care, 33,* 755–764.

Moore, F. D. (1995). *A miracle and a privilege: Recounting a half century of surgical advance.* Washington, DC: Joseph Henry Press.

Moray, N. (1994). Error reduction as a systems problem. In M. S. Bogner (Ed.), *Human Error in Medicine* (pp. 67–91). Hillsdale, NJ: Lawrence Erlbaum Associates.

Nattinger, A. B., Hoffmann, R. G., Shapiro, R., Gottlieb, M. S., & Goodwin, J. S. (1996). The effect of legislative requirements on the use of breast-conserving surgery. *New England Journal of Medicine, 335,* 1035–1040.

Orentlicher, D. (1994). The limits of legislation. *Maryland Law Review, 53,* 1255–1305.

Orient, J. M. (1994, October 6). Where new health reform should start. *Wall Street Journal,* p. A18.

Pathman, D., & Tropman, S. (1995). Obstetrical practice among new rural family physicians. *Journal of Family Practice, 40,* 457–464.

Patton, J. (1992, January 13). Quoted in *American Medical News,* p. 27.

Pauly, M. V. (1995). Practice guidelines: Can they save money? Should they? *Journal of Law, Medicine & Ethics, 23,* 65–74.

Perry, S., & Lehrman, D. (1987). Defensive medicine, malpractice, and patient satisfaction. In M. Shanahan (Ed.), *Proceedings of an international symposium on quality assurance in health care*. Chicago: Joint Commission on Accreditation of Hospitals.

Peters, J. D., Nord, S. K., & Woodson, R. D. (1986). An empirical analysis of the medical and legal professions' experiences and perceptions of medical and legal malpractice. *University of Michigan Journal of Law Reform, 19*, 601–636.

Philips, M. (1994, November). The patient's right not to know. *Johns Hopkins Magazine, 46*, 3.

Physician Payment Review Commission. (1994). *Annual report to Congress*. Washington, DC: U.S. Government Printing Office.

Piper, A., Jr. (1994). Truce on the battlefield: A proposal for a different approach to medical informed consent. *Journal of Law, Medicine & Ethics, 22*, 301–313.

Putterman, C., & Ben-Chetrit, E. (1995). Testing, testing, testing . . . . *New England Journal of Medicine, 333*, 1208–1211.

Reid, M. C., Lachs, M. S., & Feinstein, A. R. (1995). Use of methodological standards in diagnostic test research: Getting better but still not good. *Journal of the American Medical Association, 274*, 645–651.

Relman, A. (1989). The National Leadership Commission's health care plan. *New England Journal of Medicine, 320*, 314–315.

Reynolds, R. A., Rizzo, J. A., & Gonzalez, M. L. (1987). The cost of medical professional liability. *Journal of the American Medical Association, 257*, 2776–2781.

Ritchie, J. H., & Davies, S. C. (1995). Professional negligence: A duty of candid disclosure? *British Medical Journal, 310*, 888–889.

Rosoff, A. J. (1994). Truce on the battlefield: A proposal for a different approach to medical informed consent [Commentary]. *Journal of Law, Medicine & Ethics, 22*, 314–317.

Schneider, C. E. (1996, November–December). Moral discourse, bioethics, and the law. *Hastings Center Report, 26*, 37–39.

Schuck, P. H. (1994). Rethinking informed consent. *Yale Law Journal, 103*, 899–959.

Schwartz, B., Fries, S., Fitzgibbon, A. M., & Lipman, H. (1994). Pediatricians' diagnostic approach to pharyngitis and impact of CLIA 1988 on office diagnostic tests. *Journal of the American Medical Association, 271*, 234–238.

Senders, J. W. (1994). Medical devices, medical errors, and medical accidents. In M. S. Bogner (Ed.), *Human error in medicine* (pp. 159–177). Hillsdale, NJ: Lawrence Erlbaum Associates.

Shuman, D. W. (1994). The psychology of compensation in tort law. *Kansas Law Review, 43*, 39–77.

Shuman, D. W. (1993a). The psychology of deterrence in tort law. *Kansas Law Review, 42*, 115–168.

Shuman, D. W. (1993b). Making the world a better place through tort law: Through the therapeutic looking glass. *New York Law School Journal of Human Rights, 10*, 739–758.

Shuman, D. W. (1992). Therapeutic jurisprudence and tort law: A limited subjective standard of care. *Southern Methodist University Law Review, 46*, 409–432.

Siegler, M. (1975). Pascal's wager and the hanging of crepe. *New England Journal of Medicine, 293,* 853–857.

Sloan, F. A., Whetten-Goldstein, K., Githens, P. B., & Entman, S. S. (1995). Effects of the threat of medical malpractice litigation and other factors on birth outcomes. *Medical Care, 33,* 700–714.

Snyder, L., & Brennan, T. A. (1996). Disclosure of errors and the threat of malpractice. In L. Snyder (Ed.), *Ethical choices: Case studies for medical practice.* Philadelphia: American College of Physicians.

Tancredi, L. R., & Barondess, J. A. (1978). The problem of defensive medicine. *Science, 200,* 879–882.

Tenery, R. M., Jr. (1995, February 13). Should we physicians tell our patients everything? *American Medical News,* 18.

Tussing, A. D., & Wojtowycz, M. A. (1997). Malpractice, defensive medicine, and obstetric behavior. *Medical Care, 35,* 172–191.

U.S. Congress, Office of Technology Assessment. (1994). *Defensive medicine and medical malpractice.* OTA-H-602. Washington, DC: U.S. Government Printing Office.

U.S. Congress, Office of Technology Assessment. (1993). *Impact of legal reforms on medical malpractice costs.* OTA-BP-H-119. Washington, DC: U.S. Government Printing Office.

U.S. Department of Health and Human Services. (1987). *Report of the task force on medical liability and malpractice.* Washington, DC: U.S. Government Printing Office.

U.S. General Accounting Office. (1995a). *Medical liability: Impact on hospital and physician costs extends beyond insurance.* GAO/AIMD-95-169. Washington, DC.

U.S. General Accounting Office. (1995b). *VA health care: Trends in malpractice claims can aid in addressing quality of care problems.* GAO/HEHS-96-24. Washington, DC.

Verrilli, D., & Welch, G. (1996). The impact of diagnostic testing on therapeutic interventions. *Journal of the American Medical Association, 275,* 1189–1191.

Wachsman, H. F. (1993). *Lethal medicine: The epidemic of medical malpractice in America.* New York: Henry Holt and Company.

Weiler, P. C., Hiatt, H. H., Newhouse, J. P., Johnson, W. G., Brennan, T. A., & Leape, L. L. (1993). *A measure of malpractice: Medical injury, malpractice litigation, and patient compensation.* Cambridge, MA: Harvard University Press.

Weisman, C. S., Morlock, L. L., Teitelbaum, M. A., Klassen, A. C., & Celentano, D. D. (1989). Practice changes in response to the malpractice litigation climate: Results of a Maryland physician survey. *Medical Care, 27,* 16–24.

Wennberg, D. E., Kellett, M. A., Dickens, J. D., Jr., Malenka, D. J., Keilson, L. M., & Keller, R. B. (1996). The association between local diagnostic testing intensity and invasive cardiac procedures. *Journal of the American Medical Association, 275,* 1161–1164.

Witman, A. B., Park, D. M., & Hardin, S. B. (1996). How do patients want physicians to handle mistakes? A survey of internal medicine patients in an academic setting. *Archives of Internal Medicine, 156,* 2565–2569.

Wolfe, S. M. (1991). Medical ethics: A broader definition. *Mount Sinai Journal of Medicine, 58*, 455–461.

Yohai, R. A., Bullock, J. D., & Margolis, J. H. (1993). Unilateral optic disk edema and a contralateral temporal fossa mass. *American Journal of Ophthalmology, 115*, 261–262.

Risk Managers and Legal Counsel: Ethical Enablers or Paid Paranoids?

In the last two decades, the risk management profession has become an integral and accepted, indeed an expected, component of complex health care organizations (Harpster & Veach, 1990). Risk management departments and programs have proliferated during this time. The American Society for Healthcare Risk Management has become a major membership affiliate of the American Hospital Association (AHA). Specialized training and degree programs and certification opportunities are available for professional risk managers, most of whom have a nursing or other clinical background.

As exemplified by another AHA affiliate, the American Academy of Hospital Attorneys (AAHA), legal counsel also have been fruitful and multiplied within most of today's health care organizations of significant size. The particularized respective roles of the risk manager and the in-house legal counsel vary substantially among different health care facilities and agencies, as does the relationship between these two functions. For purposes of this chapter, risk managers and in-house legal counsel will be lumped together on the basis of their common interest in protecting the health care provider against avoidable legal and/or financial loss. Thus, except where noted otherwise, use here of the term risk managers is intended to include in-house legal counsel as well.

Despite the growing ubiquitousness of risk managers, most physicians claim not to feel any safer legally than they did before risk managers began to populate the health care landscape. This chapter delves into why physician anxiety has not been calmed, the ways in which physician behavior is influenced negatively and/or positively by risk managers, and some potential strategies for improving the relationship between risk managers and physicians in ways that should benefit the patient.

DO PHYSICIANS CARE WHAT RISK MANAGERS SAY?

Coming from a general background of extreme aversion to, bordering on zero tolerance of, any degree of legal risk to themselves, physicians make widely varying claims about the extent to which they and their colleagues are influenced by risk managers in actual practice. Many physicians acknowledge that how they envision the role of, and react to, risk managers depends largely on the unique culture and philosophical environment pervading one's particular health care setting; in the words of one person, the influence of risk managers is "all over the place." Organizational culture and environment, especially tangible and symbolic signals sent by governance and administration, affect the way in which risk managers define their own roles and how that role definition is projected to and interpreted by physicians within that organization. As one physician stated (although I have heard others disagree with this assessment), "The reasonable risk managers get listened to, and the paranoid ones don't." A related factor is the tremendous diversity in personalities and perspectives among particular risk managers. Physician attitudes also are influenced strongly by the individual's own prior experiences, if any, in dealing with a specific risk manager.

Some physicians, at least within certain organizations, regularly seek out and pay attention to their risk manager's advice. There are two main motivations for such physician conduct: (a) a positive attitude toward risk management's potential contribution to good patient care (discussed later) and, more frequently, (b) fear of the consequences of ignoring or disobeying the risk manager.

As an example of the latter reason, some physicians feel legally insecure enough that they routinely seek the risk manager's prior approval before engaging in innovative forms of patient treatment. Regardless of the particular question posed, after a physician has approached the risk manager for advice, he or she ordinarily feels tightly bound by the risk manager's answer and insecure in deviating from it.

Many physicians are quite aware of their own relative legal ignorance and assume, by contrast, that "risk managers must know what they are talking about." Especially when a provider organization has suffered through its own "bad case" recently, the authority of the risk manager tends to be elevated in the eyes of governance and administration, and this message gets transmitted, expressly or implicitly, to the medical staff.

However, it is likely that most physicians purposefully avoid contact with their organizational risk managers as much as possible. There may be several explanations for the extremely limited nature of the usual physician-risk manager interaction.

First, physicians tend not to initiate proactive contacts with risk managers both because physicians, according to some within as well as outside the medical profession, "are rarely proactive about anything" and because they view risk management as a function designed "to clean up existing messes." In a different but related vein, some physicians eschew anticipatory risk management because they usually operate within a state of "legal denial," that is, telling themselves, "Nothing can happen to me if I just do my best." These physicians assume that they intuitively know how to manage risk, "until the situation blows up in our face." As a corollary, those physicians who lack such a level of legal self-confidence are the ones most likely to accept risk managers' opinions as gospel.

Third, physicians are reluctant to "open up a can of worms," due to apprehension that invoking the risk manager's involvement in a case may lead to an investigation of the involved physician(s). In other words, many physicians perceive the risk management function as punitive or at least potentially so. Fourth, because few physicians (other than, sometimes, medical staff leaders) feel secure in disregarding or challenging risk managers' advice, many avoid asking questions in the first place because they anticipate difficulty in living with the excessively conservative answers (see later discussion) they believe they would be likely to receive in response to their inquiries. This anxiety leads to what several physicians described as a tacit "Don't ask, don't tell" pact among members of the medical staff and, at least for certain kinds of situations containing especially troubling ethical dilemmas, between physicians and risk managers. Indeed, some physicians only voluntarily consult risk managers when they need leverage because a patient or family is trying to prevent the physician from treating in what he or she feels is the optimal manner.

A substantial number of other physicians fail to interact proactively with risk managers not out of any conscious avoidance plan, but simply because they feel risk managers are irrelevant (i.e., "invisible" and/or unhelpful) to their daily activities. It "doesn't occur" to most physicians to consult risk managers with any regularity. As one primary care physician summed up the idea, "Legal and ethical issues are not like gastrointestinal problems, for which physicians are thoroughly trained to consult with experts."

POSITIVE PERCEPTIONS OF RISK MANAGEMENT

To the extent that physicians believe they are affected by risk management activities, for a minority that impact is characterized as positive. For practitioners in this category, their own risk managers are seen as a comforting, calming resource for information and support whom they and their fellow physicians generally underutilize.

Some physicians evaluate the inclusion of a minimum amount of risk management curriculum in continuing medical education programs in laudatory terms. A few states (namely, Massachusetts and Florida) legally mandate this educational approach. For these individuals, the preventative goals of risk management have come through clearly in educational programs that teach lawsuit reduction techniques that are useful in practice in reducing physician anxiety levels. Programs rated highly are those that convey not only potential problems but also strategies for prevention and resolution. Conversely, risk management education forays that try to capture physician attention by scaring them just counterproductively reinforce the pervasive adversarial environment.

NEGATIVE PERCEPTIONS OF RISK MANAGEMENT

The majority of physicians, though, usually are considerably less complimentary about risk managers and their influence. Sentiments such as "They're a pain" are common, as are terms like "scaredy-cats," "naysayers," "interference," and "paralysis." Most physicians ascribe to risk managers the effect of fanning, rather than alleviating, the flames of law-related anxiety for several reasons.

Risk Managers Do Not Work for the Physician

First, virtually all physicians are acutely sensitive to the risk manager's status, and hence responsibilities and loyalties, as an employee of the health care organization or institution rather than as an employee of the medical staff. Put more bluntly, physicians are quite aware that "risk managers don't work for us [physicians]." Moreover, physicians understand that most risk managers' exclusive role for their respective corporations is avoidance of legal and/or financial risk. Indeed, most risk managers make their loyalties well-known, and those who pretend to be physician or patient advocates arguably are unethically misrepresenting themselves and destroying any credibility they might have with physicians who know better than to believe such misrepresentations.

Risk Managers Are Overly Conservative

Second, risk managers are virtually unanimously criticized by physicians as overly conservative and too cautious, with a strong propensity to exaggerate risks to physicians in order to intimidate them into compliance with risk management dictates. A large number of physicians echo sentiments expressed in a book chapter entitled "Bureaucrats at the Bedside: Risk Management" (Macklin, 1993, pp. 52–76), that risk managers' narrow focus on organizational protection, at almost any cost, makes risk managers inherently anti-patient in their interests.

Many physicians, therefore, feel that risk managers practicing "defensive law" (Weisbord, 1986) force them to practice "bad medicine" on their patients, primarily by fomenting a culture in which "doing more" is always better in terms of surviving external scrutiny. This culture thereby encourages the excessive use of risky and expensive diagnostic tests and debatably therapeutic interventions. In practice, the traditional ethical admonition *Primum non nocere* frequently gets translated into, "Do no harm *unless* a lawyer [or risk manager] advises it" (Barnett, 1991, p. 410).

There is widespread medical sentiment that, as a result of this culture: (a) patients often are harmed by undergoing unnecessary risks, emotional upset, inconvenience, and expense; (b) physicians must violate their own sense of ethical commitment to principles of beneficence and nonmaleficence by harming their patients through excessive interventions; and (c) ironically, the organizational provider and its medical staff may be more exposed to liability anyway because many of the actions recommended in the name of risk management are actually counterproductive.

Physicians consistently cite two areas in which excessively conservative risk-management advice constantly impinges on good medical practice and optimal patient welfare. One sphere is that of organ harvesting for transplantation purposes. Under the Uniform Anatomical Gift Act, there exists unequivocal legal clarity in every state today that if a mentally capable individual, while alive, grants permission for organ donation to occur at the time of his or her death, no further permission is necessary to harvest the designated organ(s). Nonetheless, risk managers routinely advise health care institutions to devise and follow policies requesting permission from available family members even in such cases; institutions uniformly comply with that advice and hence obey family refusals that both disparage the autonomy of the would-be donor and tragically condemn to avoidable deaths patients who could have benefited from the numerous organs that thus become unavailable.

A second example of the disparity between risk management advice as interpreted by medical staff, on one hand, and physicians' conceptions about good patient care, on the other, is that of technological overtreatment of seriously ill and dying patients. In a survey of physicians published in 1995, for instance, 5 percent of responding physicians claimed that they had refused to honor requests by mentally capable patients to withdraw life-prolonging mechanical ventilation solely because hospital legal counsel had demurred (Asch, Hansen-Flaschen, & Lanken, 1995). This serious problem of excessive intervention near the end of life commands separate analysis in the next chapter.

The excessive conservatism exhibited by most risk managers may be a result of what some physicians perceive to be a lack of appreciation on the part of many risk managers about the realities of medical practice. Physicians frequently accuse risk managers of attempting to force patient care into an unreasonable "cookbook" mode. Additionally, some physicians make the claim that many risk managers have very underdeveloped, unsophisticated skills for resolving problems—especially those entailing patient-family-physician conflicts—informally as they unfold; this contrasts with risk managers' perceived excellent skills for dealing formally with problems after they have emerged. Whereas some physicians suggest that many risk managers' grounding in the relevant patient care law itself is weak, the bulk of negative comments center on the perceived ineptitude of many risk managers to apply the letter of the law to the everyday tangible practice of medicine. This gap between theory and realistic implementation "turns off" many physicians toward risk managers.

Unfortunately, a significant number of physicians lack the ability to distinguish between sensible, rational risk management advice and advice that is unrealistic and unnecessarily inflexible. Indeed, because most physicians are firmly inclined to think the worst of the American legal system and everything connected to it, the risk management advice that overstates potential exposure to liability the most and that paints the bleakest picture of the malpractice lottery is precisely what best catches the medical staff's attention and inspires the most vigorous, unquestioning physician compliance with whatever the risk manager commands.

Risk Managers Do Not Communicate Effectively with Physicians

Part of the problem may be that a job candidate's possession of the skills needed to communicate important legal concepts and practices effectively to physicians ordinarily is not the paramount factor in health organizations' hiring decisions for risk management positions. Consequently, these skills may often be found wanting in the persons who get those jobs.

Taking this line of criticism further, because "most physicians can't tell the difference between accurate risk management advice and nonsense," the most flamboyant risk management presentations and publications tend to make the most lasting impressions on physician audiences. More thoughtful, nuanced, and balanced analyses of issues and tactics tend to be ignored exactly because their tone is calmer. Thus, risk managers with the most constructive messages may be the messengers with the least real impact on physician behavior.

STRATEGIES FOR IMPROVING RISK MANAGER–PHYSICIAN RELATIONSHIPS

The difficulties outlined thus far are not instantly or easily solvable. It may be propitious at this time nevertheless to begin to identify some potential strategies for improving physician perceptions of risk managers, with the goal of influencing physician behavior in ways that are most consistent with organizational goals, physician interests, and patient welfare.

Initially, we must separate out erroneous physician perceptions about risk managers from those impressions that are accurate. Incorrect physician perceptions may be addressed through myriad kinds of communication and educational efforts. Risk managers and institutional/ agency administrators should establish or fortify regular channels for unambiguously informing medical staff members about the roles, goals, and processes of the risk management program within their respective organizations. Physicians within the organization should be encouraged, individually and collectively, to take advantage of constructive risk management resources.

Perhaps more importantly, it behooves risk managers to honestly examine the negative perceptions of them entertained by many physicians that, in whole or part, have a core of accuracy. As a start, risk managers should clarify their own role definitions within their respective organizations and should communicate those definitions honestly to medical staffs. To the extent that loyalty to the employing organization's legal safety trumps the risk manager's commitment to physician or patient interests, the risk manager's credibility with physicians will be enhanced by open admission of that loyalty and candid discussion of potential conflicts—as well as the substantial overlap—among the interests of the different actors providing and receiving services within the organization.

To the extent that communication barriers between risk management and the medical staff are present, they need to be identified and examined. Many risk managers may need to develop or hone specific skills that are central to effectively satisfy the unique informational needs of medical practitioners, in both large group and individual consultation settings.

Risk managers ought to examine the factual validity of physicians' characterization of most risk managers as unduly cautious and conservative, whose advice and policies often lead to practices that are clinically and ethically dubious as well as legally and financially counterproductive. To the extent that these allegations are accurate, the risk management profession through pertinent professional organizations and insurers needs to initiate one or more large-scale projects to critically evaluate its own philosophy, attitudes, and practices. This should be done with an eye toward developing and disseminating strategies that broaden and "humanize" the risk management enterprise while conscientiously fulfilling its obligations to the health care organizations and insurers who employ and sponsor risk managers in the first place.

There must be an atmosphere promoted within health care organizations that encourages physicians to seek out the risk manager's advice rather than to purposefully avoid it out of fear that it will unreasonably and inflexibly impinge on the physician's ability to practice properly. A positive atmosphere must include the opportunity for physicians to probe the rationales and authority for risk management advice that strikes them as unreasonable or otherwise ill-advised, without the risk manager becoming unduly defensive. Legal risks, like those in medicine, often are subject to numerous uncertainties; unfortunately, most risk managers are no better at dealing with their uncertainties than are physicians at dealing with theirs. (See Chapter 1 for a discussion of how physicians handle medical uncertainty poorly.) The sort of open environment in which uncertainties and honest differences of opinion can be acknowledged usually facilitates both the education of medical staff about legal probabilities and the shared negotiation of more acceptable strategies for handling potentially troubling patient care situations.

Finally (although this enumeration of strategies in no way purports to be comprehensive), physician consultations with risk managers as well as educational activities initiated by the risk management department must occur on a regular, prospective basis. Risk managers must respond to physician perceptions that risk management's influence is limited because physicians see it only as an after-the-fact, mistake-fixing and blame-apportioning operation when things have gone wrong. Risk managers must convey the message that they are a vital part of the organization's larger total quality assurance or improvement effort. The claims-management and problem-assessing functions of risk management are imperative, but the positive anticipatory, preventative purposes of proactive risk management must be emphasized as well, particularly to the medical staff constituency.

ETHICS COMMITTEES AND RISK MANAGERS

Just as risk management programs and in-house legal counsel have become abundant in health care settings over the past twenty years, so too have various versions of bioethics committees (Hoffmann, Boyle, & Levenson, 1995). Although they take various shapes and forms, these evolving entities have all been created to help health care organizations deal with difficult ethical challenges that they currently encounter or that they anticipate facing in the future. The primary functions of these interdisciplinary entities include organizational policy formulation and/or review, staff and public education, and individual case consultations. Among the most powerful factors encouraging the development of the bioethics committee mechanism in recent years have been several well-publicized judicial opinions (*In re Quinlan*, 1976), the controversy in the early 1980s surrounding federal Baby Doe regulations pertaining to medical treatment of severely handicapped newborns, 45 Code of Federal Regulations § 1340.15, Congressional enactment of the Patient Self-Determination Act as part of the 1990 Omnibus Budget Reconciliation Act, state legislation pertaining to advance medical directives and family empowerment to make medical decisions for incapacitated relatives, and new hospital standards promulgated by the Joint Commission on Accreditation of Healthcare Organizations. At least two states (Maryland and New Jersey) legally require hospitals to have ethics committees in operation (Hoffmann, 1991).

Bioethics committees have many proponents, who argue that this structure for ethical analysis conveys the advantages of objectivity, a sharing of responsibility, a broad representation of complementary professional and lay perspectives, and—last but by no means least—a degree of legal protection for the organization and its medical and other professional staff. Skeptics and critics of bioethics committees suggest, among other things, that an obsession with this last cited benefit, namely, risk management, is precisely the problem. They assert that single-mindedly concentrating on the likely benefit of legal protection often drives the actual dynamics of a committee's operation to sacrifice serious attention to truly ethical concerns. Put more directly, skeptics maintain that supposed "bioethics" committees are so only nominally, and that more often than not they quickly get perverted into quasi-risk management bodies, providing "ethical cover" or aura to impress external observers but producing little of real ethical value.

The vast majority of physicians likely fall into the skeptic category. First, physicians are even less likely to voluntarily invoke bioethics committee involvement regarding one of their patients than to seek out advice from the risk manager or in-house legal counsel. One probable reason for this reluctance is the physician's embarrassment to be "exposed" to medical peers sitting on the bioethics committee as unable to unilaterally resolve all problematic aspects of every clinical case. According to one expert speaking at a national conference on "Ethics Consultation 1996: The State of the Art," "Many, mostly physicians, think that the request for an ethics consult is an accusatory action" (Phillips, 1996, p. 1866, quoting Joel Frader, M.D.).

Moreover, as noted previously, the bioethics committee is valued by physicians primarily as a mechanism for achieving an externally acceptable ethical stamp of approval that conveys a patina of legal prophylaxis, rather than for its ability to identify and parse out perplexing ethical dilemmas through an ethically appropriate process. Thus, a physician who receives objectionable advice from a bioethics committee often will then consult with the organizational risk manager in the hope of receiving contrary advice that is more consistent with the physician's preconceived notion of the best result.

Some physicians who serve as members of bioethics committees complain that, at their worst, overly conservative risk managers can rapidly disrupt the salutary effects of education and consultation provided by bioethics committees to medical staffs. When there is a conflict between advice tendered by a bioethics committee or other ethics consultant, on one hand, and that urged by risk management, on the other, physicians almost uniformly (albeit unenthusiastically and sometimes reluctantly) err on the risk manager's side.

The perverse conversion of bioethics committees into *de facto* (or at least believed to be) risk management mechanisms is nicely, even if probably unintentionally and in a somewhat exaggerated manner, exemplified in philosopher Brendan Minogue's recent book on hospital bioethics committees (Minogue, 1996; Mitchell, 1997). In the context of a hypothetical bioethics committee's consideration of a case, Minogue describes John Quinn, a caricature of a hospital attorney serving on the bioethics committee but who is concerned solely with conjecturing about the hospital's theoretical exposure to litigation and legal liability and who was virtually disdainful of the case's ethical dimensions.

Quinn's first question, after hearing that the patient has contacted the bioethics committee to complain about allegedly inadequate informed consent, is "Has the patient hired counsel to represent him?" (p. 127). Later in the same case, attorney Quinn complains, "I signed on to this committee to assist at the level of ethics policy development and consultation. I did not wish to get involved in evaluating specific people" (Minogue, 1996, p. 131). In a subsequent discussion of a potential surrogacy arrangement, he is challenged by one of the physician committee members, who asks him whether he is "playing the role of hospital attorney or the role of a member of the committee," because the physician is concerned about the "possible conflict of interest" (p. 181). Quinn replies, "My expertise is in the area of law, risk management, and liability. That is what I know very well. I think surrogacy is still legally uncharted territory and poses possible risk to the hospital. I feel we should avoid it" (p. 181).

CONCLUSION

One outspoken critic of risk managers' influence on the quality of patient care and medical ethics has written:

> Risk management must be balanced by patient advocacy. . . . If legal consultants and other risk managers find that good care must be compromised to minimize institutional risk, then they need to make this fact known publicly both to the people being admitted to their facility, and to the legislators and reviewers who have generated these well-intended but ultimately harmful policies. (Quill, 1993)

Quill's view of the dynamics at work here is pessimistic indeed, but it usefully raises a red flag of concern. Risk management advice that is perceived as conflicting with sound clinical precepts, accepted ethical principles, humane treatment of persons, and the just and reasonable allocation of scarce resources is counterproductive in that it breeds distrust and disrespect for risk management and for the legal system. It drives conduct underground, into hiding and silence, or causes decisions to be made by inaction or default. Advice that fails to command commitment weakens respect for the legitimate risk management guidance that should be taken seriously as the basis for decisions and actions.

Ideally, the growing involvement of risk managers and in-house legal counsel within modern health care settings ought to add to, rather than detract from, physicians' capacity to provide ethically acceptable medical care to patients. The humanization of medicine demands that strategies be developed and implemented to enhance and magnify the salutary role these actors could play and to rectify the perverse influences they often currently exert.

REFERENCES

Asch, D. A., Hansen-Flaschen, J., & Lanken, P. N. (1995). Decisions to limit or continue life-sustaining treatment by critical care physicians in the United States: Conflicts between physicians' practices and patients' wishes. *American Journal of Respiratory Critical Care Medicine, 151*, 288–292.

Barnett, T. J. (1991). Lawyer's advice [Letter]. *Annals of Internal Medicine, 115*, 409–410.

Harpster, L. M., & Veach, M. S. (Eds.). (1990). *Risk management handbook for health care facilities.* Chicago, IL: American Hospital Publishing.

Hoffmann, D. E. (1991). Does legislating hospital ethics committees make a difference? A study of hospital ethics committees in Maryland, the District of Columbia, and Virginia. *Law, Medicine and Health Care, 19*, 105–119.

Hoffmann, D. E., Boyle, P., & Levenson, S. A. (1995). *Handbook for nursing home ethics committees.* Washington, DC: American Association of Homes and Services for the Aging.

In re Quinlan (1976), 70 N.J. 10, 355 A.2d 647, *cert. denied*, 429 U.S. 922.

Macklin, R. (1993). *Enemies of patients.* New York: Oxford University Press.

Minogue, B. (1996). *Bioethics: A committee approach.* Sudbury, MA: Jones and Bartlett Publishers.

Mitchell, S. M. (1997). Book review of *Bioethics: A Committee Approach* by B. Minogue. *Journal of Ethics, Law, and Aging, 3*(1), 62–66.

Phillips, D. F. (1996). Ethics consultation quality: Is evaluation feasible? *Journal of the American Medical Association, 275*, 1866–1867.

Quill, T. E. (1993). *Death and dignity: Making choices and taking charge.* New York: W.W. Norton & Company.

Weisbord, A. J. (1986). Defensive law: A new perspective on informed consent. *Archives of Internal Medicine, 146*, 860–861.

4

Doing Everything: Treating Legal Fears near the End of Life

A firm legal (Meisel, 1992) and ethical (Hastings Center, 1987) position has developed in the United States over the past quarter century in favor of shared medical decision making, including but not limited to (Wolf & Becker, 1996) decisions regarding the critically ill and dying. This position is premised on a process of communication and negotiation over time taking place among the mentally capable patient, family members and significant friends, physician, and other members of the health care team (President's Commission, 1982; Cummins, 1992; Miller, Coe, & Hyers, 1992). Such a process best embodies the important value of individual patient autonomy (Gauthier, 1993).

Recent studies have scientifically documented through health services research techniques what health care providers, patients, and families have long known by instinct and personal observation (Quill, 1995)—namely, that medical care near the end of life too often deviates widely from the clinical, emotional, and indeed ethical ideal. In the early 1990s, the Robert Wood Johnson Foundation headquartered in Princeton, New Jersey, lavishly funded the Study to Understand Prognosis and Preferences for Outcomes and Risks of Treatment (SUPPORT), designed to increase understanding of the process of hospitalized dying and to devise interventions—that is, improved communications, clarification and coordination of patient and family preferences, and pain control—to promote more humane and compassionate care. A careful multicenter evaluation of their impact proved conclusively that these interventions failed miserably to achieve their goals (SUPPORT Principal Investigators, 1995). The results of the SUPPORT study were entirely consistent with those reported in previous evaluations (Danis, Southerland, Garrett, Smith, Hielema, Pickard, et al., 1991; Schneiderman, Kronick, Kaplan, Anderson, & Langer, 1992; Teno, Lynn, & Phillips, 1994), as well as subsequent ones (Jacobson, Kasworm, Battin, Francis, Green, Botkin, et al., 1996; Tonelli, 1996).

The continued ethical deficiencies in the delivery of end-of-life care even in the face of precisely the sorts of humanistic strategies that have been urged for years raise a host of questions (Moskowitz & Nelson, 1995; Snider, 1995) and implicate a variety of culprits (Lynn, 1996). At least one of those culprits is the law (McCrary, Swanson, Perkins, & Winslade, 1992). Law Professor George Annas (1978) has described the modern American attitude toward dying within the health care system as follows:

> Death is a natural process and a uniquely personal experience. If pressed to categorize it, most would probably term the major controversies surrounding it ethical, rather than medical or legal. Nevertheless, there is an increasing trend to ask the courts whether life-sustaining treatment should be withheld from patients who are unable to make this decision themselves. Judges are asked to decide this question, not because they have any special expertise, but because only they can provide the physicians with civil and criminal immunity for their actions. In seeking this immunity, legal considerations quickly transcend ethical and medical judgments. (p. 21)

Though Annas in this quote substantially overstates the degree to which courts become involved in end-of-life decision making, provider perception of the legal system continually lurking in the shadows is both real and powerful (Mondragon, 1987). As put by one physician discussing end-of-life medical decision making, "Any physician who has been in this situation before would readily admit that these legal issues [pertaining to the physician's own potential liability] do weigh heavily on a decision of this type" (Griffin, 1997).

The negative influence of defensive medicine on the clinical, emotional, and even ethical quality of care near the end of patients' lives has been much lamented. For example, physician Timothy Quill (1992, p. 495) has observed that end-of-life decision making frequently is "influenced more by considerations of risk management than by those of patient care," and philosopher Daniel Callahan (1993, p. 39) notes, "A worry about malpractice . . . [as well as several other factors] often lead to overtreatment and an excessive reliance on technology." Over a decade ago, an influential group of physicians well familiar with issues surrounding the withholding and withdrawal of life-sustaining medical treatment (LSMT) wrote, "Fear of legal liability often interferes with the physician's ability to make the best choice for the patient" (Wanzer, Adelstein, Cranford, Federman, Hook, Moertel, et al., 1984, p. 955).

That fear persists still. Clearly, no one today wants to be asked, "Who was responsible for this patient's death?"

Too many of today's physicians caring for seriously ill and dying patients feel themselves compelled by institutional policies and risk management directives to initiate and continue aggressive life-prolonging medical interventions in situations where clinical and ethical considerations—and frequently also the wishes of the patient and/or surrogates—argue for withholding or withdrawing various forms of intervention (Lo & Steinbrook, 1991; Dubler, 1993). Whether this belief is correct or erroneous matters little in a practical sense. Although many physicians characterize the present state of medical practice at the end of life as "overkill," ironically, "overlife" might be a more apt label. Physicians who order abatement of maximum aggressive medical assaults when they believe the real burdens outweigh any speculative benefits for the patient often feel they are taking a real gamble with liability in order to do the "right thing" (Quill, 1994). Instead of taking this perceived gamble, many physicians (between 30 and 40 percent in one study [Solomon, O'Donnell, Jennings, Guilfoy, Wolf, Nolan, et al., 1993]) recognize the law/ethics tension but admit to acting contrary to their consciences by overtreating dying patients because of liability threats (Wynia, 1994).

EXAMPLES OF LEGISOGENIC INAPPROPRIATE TREATMENT NEAR THE END OF LIFE

Legally induced (I would suggest the term "legisogenic") medically inappropriate treatment near the end of life takes several specific forms. In different cases, it may be manifested as too much or too little medical intervention, especially for very young (Harvard Law Review Staff, 1990, pp. 1584–1614) or very old patients.

A paradigm illustration of the terrible human impact of this sort of risk management–induced physician mentality may be found in the notorious *Linares* case that occurred in a Chicago neonatal intensive care unit in 1989. There, the father of a severely and irreversibly brain-damaged infant diagnosed as persistently vegetative who had swallowed a balloon became distraught at the physician's refusal to withdraw life-prolonging mechanical ventilation from the infant, due to the physician feeling bound to continue treatment by excessively conservative advice received from the hospital's in-house counsel. In frustration, Mr. Linares held the hospital's medical and nursing staffs hostage with a gun while he disconnected the equipment himself and his son expired (Nelson & Cranford, 1989).

In another neonatal case, physician Gregory Messenger was charged with manslaughter for physically disconnecting his premature son from a ventilator after the attending physicians refused, and he was acquitted by a jury (Clark, 1996). Moral paralysis resulting in excessive medical assaults on newborns stems in part (although there are differences of opinion regarding how important a factor this is [Moskop & Saldanha, 1986; Murray, 1985; Young & Stevenson, 1990]) from uncertainty about interpretation of the federal Baby Doe law, 42 United States Code §§ 5102–5106, 5111–5113, 45 Code of Federal Regulations part 1340, which makes inadequate infant care a violation of state child abuse and neglect statutes (Caplan, Blank, & Merrick, 1992).

At the other end of the age spectrum, physicians almost universally acknowledge overly aggressive infliction of LSMT interventions on elderly critically ill and dying patients, inspired by apprehension about various potential types of liability (Fried, Stein, O'Sullivan, Brock, & Novack, 1993). Even LSMT that is believed by the physician to be medically futile (Kapp, 1994) or nonbeneficial for the patient often is provided anyway—with or without (Asch, Hansen-Flaschen, & Lanken, 1995) authorized consent—in order to "treat" someone (e.g., real or contemplated demanding family members, regulators, or attorneys) other than the patient (Schneiderman & Jecker, 1995, pp. 83–96; Snider, 1995). The power to materially affect the course of a patient's treatment in this way usually bears no relationship to the particular feared non-patient's actual legal standing on behalf of the patient. Nonetheless, in what physicians perceive as the current "environment" (that is, the legal environment) (Fowkes, 1994), such legisogenically derived LSMT (Office of Technology Assessment, 1987) interventions may take several forms.

One example mentioned repeatedly in the literature and in physicians' conversations is attempts at cardiopulmonary resuscitation (CPR) on patients for whom the realistic expected benefit or chance for long-term success is negligible (Gupta, 1991). It is not difficult to figure out why CPR attempts are often inflicted on inappropriate candidates. One prominent source of misinformation in this regard was the 1983 version of an American Heart Association course on CPR that most physicians must take each year to renew hospital privileges or medical licenses. This course advised that CPR be administered to almost all cardiac arrest victims brought to the emergency room without prehospital CPR, unless an order not to resuscitate had been properly written previously by the attending physician. CPR was recommended even for patients typically designated "dead on arrival," because—physicians were told—a plaintiff's attorney may successfully contest the claim that circulatory arrest had been present for such a long time that recovery of brain function would be impossible (McIntyre, 1983).[1]

Such conservative advice suggests that the risk of malpractice litigation is so great that physicians would be prudent to attempt CPR even though it is extremely unlikely to benefit the patient. In actuality, that malpractice risk is extremely small, because overwhelming evidence of the dismal success rate of CPR attempts (Dull, Graves, Larsen, & Cummins, 1994; Murphy, Murray, Robinson, & Campion, 1989) would make it very difficult for a plaintiff's attorney to prove that the failure to provide a generally futile intervention proximately or directly caused the patient some injury.

Fears and uncertainties about potential litigation and liability also may sometimes lead physicians to make decisions about CPR out of public view, without justification or documentation of those decisions. In a study of DNR orders in San Francisco in the mid-1980s, physicians in 4 out of 136 cases gave oral orders to nurses not to resuscitate patients in case of cardiopulmonary arrest but deliberately did not write the orders in the medical records. In these 4 cases, the physicians disagreed with the families of incompetent patients about the decisions. In 6 cases, the physicians gave "limited," "slow," or "partial" code orders (Lo, Saika, Strull, Thomas, & Showstack, 1985).

Such conduct runs afoul of the ethical ideal that patient care decisions should be made and justified openly, and it ironically increases rather than diminishes the legal risk exposure for all involved health care providers. Largely as a result of the federal Patient Self-Determination Act (PSDA) enacted by Congress in 1990, Public Law No. 101-508 §§4206, 4751, requiring health care entities to develop and adopt formal written policies on matters such as CPR, as well as relevant state statutes passed in the past decade (Meisel, 1995a, pp. 555–576) and relatively recent standards on institutional CPR policies and procedures imposed by the Joint Commission on the Accreditation of Healthcare Organizations (JCAHO) (Joint Commission, 1996, § MA.1.4.11), the practices listed in the preceding paragraph have diminished greatly in incidence. Nonetheless, fear of litigation still drives a certain amount of CPR conduct underground in the hospital setting.

Legisogenically inspired inappropriate CPR attempts raise ethical objections not only within the hospital setting, though; they are a major ethical problem in prehospital situations as well. Today, many critically ill and dying persons choose to spend the last portion of their lives in their own homes or those of family members, with the notion that when it occurs, death will be a dignified event (Kapp, 1995a). Not infrequently, however, despite substantial discussion and preparation precisely intended to avoid this tragedy, when confronted with death's reality at the moment of cardiac arrest, family members panic and telephone 911 for paramedic support. When the paramedics arrive, they feel legally compelled to engage in maximum aggressive intervention, including cardiac life support, even over contemporaneous objections voiced by the patient and family.

A 1991 report (Sachs, Miles, & Levin, 1991) verified that local emergency medical system (EMS) providers identified legal concerns as a primary barrier to enacting prehospitalization Do Not Resuscitate (DNR) policies. Several EMS officials assumed (without any actual investigation of the facts) that prehospital DNR policies would require enabling state legislation to integrate such policies with existing statutes governing EMS operations more generally or advance directive laws. Other officials insisted on an explicit shield law providing EMS providers with absolute legal immunity as a precondition of abating any available form of medical treatment regardless of the predictable burden/benefit ratio.

Another mode of LSMT that frequently is motivated by legal anxieties in large part is life prolongation by artificial feeding and hydration, through nasogastric (NG) or surgically implanted percutaneous endoscopic gastrostomy (PEG) tubes (Hodges & Tolle, 1994; Major, 1986), of critically ill and dying, often permanently vegetative, patients for periods of indefinite duration. Health care facilities often force artificial feeding in ethically questionable circumstances (i.e., in the absence of voluntary and competent consent as well as a disproportionate burden/benefit ratio arguing against such treatment on best interests principles [Payne, Taylor, Stocking, & Sachs, 1996]). This is done frequently out of an exaggerated fear of being accused of nutritional neglect of patients (Parker & Buller, 1994).

To compound the ethical affront, uncomfortable and undignified physical or mechanical restraints (Moss & LaPuma, 1991) (see Chapter 5) often are ordered by the physician to prevent the patient from effectuating his or her choice to manually remove unwanted feeding tubes (Hodges, Tolle, Stocking, & Cassel, 1994). A leading geriatrician (who ought to know better) writes of his ethical quandary in a case involving a 99-year-old, severely demented, emaciated woman who would not eat by mouth:

> The burdens of tube feeding can be substantial. I'm worried about the basic ones. Will she survive the tube placement? Will restraints be needed? What effect will the increase in urine and stool have? In the eyes of the Law, these

burdens are inconsequential, and the right path is clear. If her life can be prolonged, it must be. I am not so sure. (Finucane, 1993, p. 659)

The dangers of ethically inappropriate tube feeding are especially present in the nursing home setting. There, the absence of much precedent in the form of case law, lack of good understanding of the limited precedent that does exist, and especially misinterpretation and exaggeration (by both providers and government surveyors) of the complex web of regulatory provisions (Kapp, 1995b, pp. 30–32) that engulfs nursing home care combine to inflict highly aggressive treatment on individuals for whom foreseeable burdens far exceed the negligible benefits. Even more than hospitals, nursing home personnel often feel that they must behave in this fashion; fear of being cited for nutritional neglect by state surveyors and suffering administrative sanctions accordingly, and the accompanying public sullying of the facility's reputation, is a powerful force for overtreatment.

42 Code of Federal Regulations §483.25 (i) provides:

(i) **Nutrition**. Based on a resident's comprehensive assessment, the facility must insure that a resident—
(1) Maintains acceptable parameters of nutritional status, such as body weight and protein levels, unless the resident's clinical condition demonstrates that this is not possible; and
(2) Receives a therapeutic diet when there is a nutritional problem.

42 Code of Federal Regulations §483.25 (g) provides:

(g) **Naso-gastric tubes**. Based on the comprehensive assessment of a resident, the facility must ensure that—
(1) A resident who has been able to eat enough alone or with assistance is not fed by naso-gastric tube unless the resident's clinical condition demonstrates that use of a naso-gastric tube was unavoidable; and
(2) A resident who is fed by a naso-gastric or gastrostomy tube receives the appropriate treatment and services to prevent aspiration pneumonia, diarrhea, vomiting, dehydration, metabolic abnormalities, and nasal-pharyngeal ulcers and to restore, if possible, normal eating skills.

Nursing homes also are subject to state regulations. In Pennsylvania, for instance, facilities are explicitly required to meet the daily nutritional needs of patients, 28 Pa. Code §211.6(a).

Post and Whitehouse (1995) write regarding regulations about caloric intake:

Some nursing homes are fearful of allowing a person with profound and terminal dementia to die peacefully, as they have throughout the course of history. Instead, they routinely provide artificial feeding in order to avoid possible penalties imposed by the state when residents lose weight. . . . In some cases, state inspectors are more interested in measuring weight than in taking dementia and ethics into account. (p. 1428)

Timothy Quill (1994) supports this observation. "In New York State nursing facilities," he has noted, "we have literally thousands of demented elderly people who are kept alive by feeding tubes not because people believe that is the right thing to do, but because people are legally afraid to stop them" (p. 697).

At the same time that they complain about the law compelling overtreatment of the critically ill and dying, however, many physicians also protest that they are inhibited from providing adequate analgesic treatment to dying patients in intractable pain (Desbiens, Wu, Broste, Wenger, Connors, Lynn, Yasui, Phillips, & Fulkerson, 1996; Lasch & Carr, 1996) because risk managers and/or other sources of legal information and misinformation have frightened them about potential criminal or administrative liability under federal and state controlled drug prescription laws. In a 1994 survey, eighty-three out of ninety-eight responding physicians answered affirmatively to both of the following questions:

> 1. In your opinion, has the potential for disciplinary action by your state medical board or any other agency caused physicians in your state to be more conservative (in dosage, drug choice and refills) when prescribing medications for the treatment of chronic, intractable pain?
> 2. If yes, has the potential for disciplinary action caused you to be more conservative in your prescribing to the degree that your patients may not be receiving adequate pain relief?

Another eleven physicians answered "yes" to the first question only (Skelly, 1994a, 1994b, 1994c, and 1994d). Moreover, many physicians believe that risk managers have convinced institutions to adopt internal policies and procedures restricting physicians' ability to prescribe pain-controlling agents sufficiently.

Indeed, many physicians are under the impression that they must be risking punishment when they do provide pain relief consistent with the ethical principle of beneficence (Borneman & Ferrell, 1996; van der Poel, 1996; Rouse, 1994; Longergan, 1996; Blum, Simpson, & Blum, 1990). Speaking of analgesic care, one eminent practitioner has confessed, "Like so many of my colleagues, I have more than once broken the law to ease a patient's going, because my promise, spoken or implied, could not be kept unless I did so" (Nuland, 1994, pp. 242–243). As another put it, "There is real fear of being accused of overmedicating, even where patients are dying in agonizing pain" (Quill, 1994, p. 704). The legal confusion surrounding this matter extends to Canadian physicians as well as those in the United States (Casswell, 1990).

A number of physicians believe that they and their colleagues have "tortured" (a word used by more than a few) patients by withholding pain medications in order to preserve those patients' mental capacity to consent to or refuse other forms of medical intervention. Ironically, in many cases keeping individuals in unnecessary intractable pain probably has the precise opposite effect of impairing both cognitive ability at the time and the voluntariness of any decisions. In any event, it certainly violates clinical and ethical, as well as economic, treatment principles around which there is firm consensus among medical leaders (Crowley, 1994).

The legal anxiety surrounding drug prescription for palliative purposes is not totally without some foundation (Gianelli, 1996a; Shapiro, 1994a and 1994b). In the wake of the unsuccessful but highly publicized global "war on drugs" of the past couple of decades, many states now require special prescription forms or multiple original prescriptions for certain controlled substances and limit the number of pills or the dosage that may be prescribed (Rhymes, 1996, p. 408). Such cumbersome administrative requirements effectively discourage physicians from bothering with these medications (Behr, 1994).

A closely related, although separable, issue from that of pain control is that of physician-assisted suicide, that is, active physician intervention (e.g., prescribing a drug overdose or hooking up the patient to a lethal machine that the patient can activate by flipping a switch or giving a voice command) done with the intention and expectation of hastening the patient's death rather than letting nature take its course (Fins, 1996). A full discussion of the legal and ethical ramifications of this topic are beyond the scope of this book (Symposium, 1996). It must be noted in this context, though, that many proponents of legalizing the practice of physician-assisted suicide on humane grounds argue that currently prevalent criminal laws are an unethical barrier to physicians' capacity to respond humanely to the small but real cohort of patients for whom no other benevolent alternative exists (Brody, 1992; Cassell, 1991). According to this view, the law is objectionable because it adds to the existing suffering by forcing the patient "to die alone" (Quill, 1993), and "We all should be troubled that laws can reinforce that kind of aloneness at the end" (Quill, 1994, p. 702).

At the same time, as noted in an excellent recent review of this subject (Cantor & Thomas, 1996),several states have exempted pain relief from the scope of criminal bans on assisted suicide. Michigan law, for example, protects use of medication designed "to relieve pain or discomfort and not to cause death, even if the medication or procedure may hasten or increase the risk of death." North Dakota has authorized "use of medications or procedures necessary to relieve a person's pain or discomfort if . . . not intentionally or knowingly prescribed or administered to cause death." Florida authorizes the use of controlled substances for intractable pain "in accordance with that level of care . . . recognized by a reasonably prudent physician." Three states implicitly authorize even risky pain relief in their officially endorsed advance directive forms that use language requesting pain relief even if it hastens death. Colorado established a task force in 1996 to examine this topic (Associated Press, 1996a).

At its 1996 Annual Meeting, the American Medical Association indicated that it would draft model legislation to ensure that physicians prescribing drugs to patients in great pain are not charged with improperly dispensing controlled substances. An AMA report said, "The failure of most states to expressly permit the practice has generated reluctance among physicians" to prescribe controlled substances for physical pain or depression (Page, 1996). Medical boards and state legislatures appear to be slowly heeding the call, as they review their existing laws and guidelines on optimal pain treatment (Gianelli, 1996b).

In addition, the AMA has created the Coalition for Quality End-of-Life Care for the purpose of fighting physician-assisted suicide by promoting better end-of-life care of persons in pain (Protecting, 1996). Founding members of this coalition are listed in Figure 4.1. Further, the American Board of Internal Medicine has initiated a project on Caring for the Dying: Identification and Promotion of Physician Competency

Figure 4.1
Founding Members of Coalition for Quality End-of-Life Care.

American Academy of Family Physicians
American Academy of Hospice and Palliative Medicine
American Academy of Pain Medicine
American Academy of Physician Assistants
American Geriatrics Society
American Medical Association
American Medical Directors Association
American Nurses Association
American Osteopathic Association
California Medical Association
Center to Improve Care of the Dying (George Washington University)
New York State Task Force on Life and the Law
Society of Critical Care Medicine

(ABIM, 1996a and 1996b). The Robert Wood Johnson Foundation has joined in this effort by funding an ambitious "Last Acts" project pulling together a number of professional groups.

Deficiencies in reimbursement methodologies also have been an important inhibitor of appropriate pain control among critically ill and dying patients. These methodologies are now beginning to be corrected (Cassel & Vladeck, 1996). It is quite possible that many physicians who presently treat pain poorly used their stated fear of litigation and legal liability as a pretext for their deficient behavior, while in reality being influenced mainly by the earlier financial disincentives to good care. Legal anxieties may also serve in this context to mask other kinds of real barriers (e.g., educational and psychological) inhibiting optimal pain management (Cleland, 1987; Bruera, Fox, Chadwick, Brenneis, & Mac-Donald, 1987; Ferrell, McCaffery, & Rhiner, 1992).

Impaired communication and interpersonal relationships with family members of critically ill and dying persons represent another area in which physicians report that legal demons exert a negative impact. For instance, in end-of-life situations some physicians are less likely to bring up certain options in discussion if they are afraid that the patient or family may misinterpret these discussions and turn them against the physician later for legal purposes; the legal specter, thus, may serve as an inhibitor to honest dialogue, support, and mutual trust just when they are most needed. In this vein, a future president of the American College of Physicians and respected expert in medical ethics testified before Congress:

> I think that the tremendously adversarial environment that the current malpractice crisis in our profession has created makes American physicians want to get a contract from their patients. So they turn the whole decision over to the family or the patient, which then makes the family feel like it is their fault that the patient died, rather than the more comforting notion of a physician who is brave enough to put her arm around someone's shoulder and say, medical science cannot keep your mother alive much longer, but she will not suffer and we will take good care of her. (Cassel, 1994, p. 7)

As often as not, legislation intended to improve the quality and ethics of medical practice near the end of life by clarifying respective legal rights and responsibilities ends up actually exerting an opposite impact (Zinberg, 1989, pp. 479–481). For example, physicians' difficulties in striving to comply with a confusing and massively overreaching New York State DNR statute, N.Y. Public Health Law §§ 2960–2979, with horrible consequences for patients, are well documented (Macklin, 1993, p. 46; McClung & Kramer, 1990).

> In New York the fear of litigation or investigation by the Health Department cannot be overestimated. Few patients facing this choice have made explicit statements, and the state has provided no definition of "reasonable knowledge" [of an incompetent patient's wishes]. Therefore, many patients now receive artificial hydration and nutrition if there is any uncertainty about their wishes, sometimes even when this overrides the substituted decision of caring families or proxies. The discrepancy between the law's intent and its implementation illustrates a danger in legislating ethics. (Quill, 1992)

Based on the findings from a survey of New York physicians about their understanding of that state's DNR order, one physician has asserted discouragingly, "Physicians may be continuing to try on a case-by-case basis to find the best path for each dying patient. When that happens in New York State it is, unfortunately, illegal" (Pollack, 1996, p. 1371).

Even when patients have executed advance directive documents (Meisel, 1995a, pp. 1–270) such as living wills and durable powers of attorney in compliance with applicable state statutes, physicians fear being more hamstrung than helped by the inherent limitations of those documents (Emanuel, 1993). Such a result is virtually inevitable given the clumsy legislative drafting and crass power politics, as opposed to intelligent and frank consideration of ethical concerns, that have shaped state advance directive legislation (Kapp, 1992).

Writing about advance directives, one set of legal scholars has suggested:

> Because the development of the statutory forms occurs in the legislative arena, their content is the result of a political rather than a "scientific" process. The forms are not tested on a random sample of consumers [or physicians]; rather, they are developed in the context of political debate. In some cases, the debate is heated, and significant controversy has arisen over the content of the forms. . . . As a result of political compromise, many of the forms ultimately passed by the legislatures are not optimal from a consumer [or physician] perspective. The forms may be difficult to understand and confusing to those attempting to complete them without assistance [or to implement them on behalf of patients]. (Hoffmann, Zimmerman, & Tompkins, 1996, pp. 5–6)

A 1995 survey of a sample of Ohio physicians documented at best a very modest positive net effect on clinicians' legal comfort, patient and family relations, and willingness to comply with ethical dictates to abate aggressive medical intervention as a result of the legislature's haphazard enactment of a makeshift advance directive and family consent statute (Kapp, 1996). In many cases, excessive medical interventions may be traced to state advance directives legislation making physicians less willing to engage in independent "prudential judgments" about the wisdom of those interventions.

A legal commentator with extensive experience observing in medical centers has summarized this situation:

> In actual practice, evidence suggests that patients' ability to have their wishes regarding the prohibition of life-sustaining treatment honored may be impeded in states where natural death legislation exists. For, if such legislation is viewed by attending physicians and healthcare providers as the sole means for both initiating and implementing a decision to forego treatment and if they maintain that a decision of this nature cannot be made by a surrogate on behalf of another but only in strict accordance with an advance directive that has been executed properly by a patient, dying patients may in fact be subject to treatment the nature of which is neither requested nor beneficial. There is additional fear that an improper inference may be drawn that if a patient has not executed a directive that is in compliance with natural death legislation, he or she does not wish methods of life-sustaining treatment to be ended under any and all circumstances. (Smith, 1996, p. 59)

Informal patient directives may be just as, if not more, ethically and legally compelling as written declarations (Sachs & Siegler, 1991).

One looking for a tangible description of the emotional hell through which one set of health care providers unethically put one family, as a consequence of slavishly following overly conservative legal advice that was based on a narrow interpretation of a rationally incomprehensible and logically inconsistent state advance directive statute, should read law professor Gere Fulton's moving account of the human aspects of the *Kramp* case that unfolded in Ohio's Lucas County Probate Court. Having served as legal advisor to the family in that case, he witnessed firsthand the moral and psychological destruction wreaked by inept legislative intrusion into intimate medical and personal affairs, as exacerbated by myopic risk management. In one of several conversations with the hospital attorney, Fulton was told (apparently with the speaker impervious to both the immediate human and the larger institutional policy implications of his statement), "[W]e're getting a heinous result, but we're doing the right [risk management] thing." Fulton (1994) could only conclude, after the court permitted the dying patient to die essentially by ignoring the Ohio statute and the hospital attorney's reading of it, "This is a tragic waste of time, energy, and money for all who are consigned to dwell in this legal wonderland" (p. 595). A description of this sort of legally induced agony has also been presented from the perspective of a patient's daughter (Hansot, 1996).

WHAT'S THE MATTER?

As the discussion thus far establishes clearly, anxiety about possible litigation and liability on the part of physicians—the fear "that anything less than [ethically] mindless continuation of aggressive treatments would make them legally vulnerable" (Schneiderman, 1994, p. 65)—and other health care providers too frequently results in ethically dubious medical treatment for critically ill and dying patients. Current or prospectively stated patient wishes may be ignored, and family wishes may be either overridden or, conversely, obeyed even when unreasonable and not in the patient's best interests (Kayser-Jones & Kapp, 1989). Why is this the case? More specifically, can we delineate with any more precision what it is that physicians et al. really fear, and from whom they fear it, should they frustrate the public's yearnings for magic and miracles?

"The legal climate . . . [that] conspires to deter physicians from limiting treatment" (Gillick, 1994, p. 174) for the critically ill and dying has three distinct but related components. Individual and institutional health care providers fear criminal prosecution, civil liability, and regulatory sanctions.

Criminal Prosecution

Physician fears of criminal prosecution for limiting life-sustaining medical interventions in the end-of-life context are an excellent example of the way in which a few isolated incidents involving unique fact patterns (*Green v. Abrams*, 1993; *People v. Anyakora*, 1993; *State v. Warden*, 1991; *People v. Coe*, 1988; *People v. Protopappas*, 1988; *State v. Brenner*, 1986; *State v. Serebin*, 1984; *People v. Cabral*, 1983; *Commonwealth v. Youngkin*, 1981; *Commonwealth v. Kominsky*, 1976; *State v. Killory*, 1976; *People v. Ketchum*, 1974) can be so overpublicized, misrepresented, and misinterpreted that serious damage can be done to the ethical practice of medicine. Although the objective risk of criminal prosecution in this particular context is extremely small (Van Grunsven, 1996; Smith, 1995), it looms large in the minds of many physicians who make and carry out treatment decisions for critically ill and dying patients (Allen, 1996).

One main culprit is the *Barber* case (1983). It arose over a decade ago, represents one of only two homicide prosecutions in American history against physicians for abating treatment of a dying patient, came to the prosecutor's attention because of a vehement public confrontation between a nurse and the attending physician, and resulted in all charges being dismissed before trial. Nonetheless, large numbers of current physicians still often cite this prosecution to justify their admittedly excessive treatment of dying patients (McCrary, Swanson, Perkins, & Winslade, 1992).

A more recent source of physician anxiety is the New York criminal prosecution of Dr. Gerald Einaugler (*People v. Einaugler*, 1994). The patient in this case was a seventy-eight-year-old demented woman with end-stage renal disease, diabetes, and cardiovascular disease. She was transferred from a hospital to a nursing facility in May 1990. At the nursing facility, Dr. Einaugler mistook the patient's peritoneal-dialysis catheter for a gastrostomy tube and directed staff to feed the patient through it. Several feedings through the dialysis catheter were provided before a nurse discovered the mistake. Dr. Einaugler consulted by phone with a nephrologist, who advised him to "get the patient into the hospital." After this conversation, Dr. Einaugler examined the patient but decided to delay the transfer. On admission ten hours later, peritonitis was diagnosed and the patient died shortly thereafter.

The delay led to prosecution. "The lynchpin of both counts is not the carelessness that caused the patient to be fed Isocal through the dialysis catheter. This error, however horrifying and incompetent, was a mistake from ignorance, not a mistake made with any criminal intent. Instead, the criminal conduct in the indictment was petitioner's failure to hospitalize the patient after he became aware." In July 1993 Dr. Einaugler was convicted of reckless endangerment of his patient and willful violation of New York's health laws and sentenced to spend a year's worth of weekends in jail. In 1994 the appeals court unanimously upheld the jury's verdict.

Despite the appeals court's calm assurance that this case "does not support the proposition that medical professionals need fear the prospect of unwarranted criminal prosecutions for honest errors of medical judgment" and academic pronouncements that "[r]esponsible physicians have nothing to fear from the criminal law" (Annas, 1995, p. 530), the reaction of practicing physicians to the Einaugler prosecution and conviction has not been sanguine. Having reviewed hundreds of letters and telephone calls from physicians, American Medical Association General Counsel Kirk Johnson observed, "What they know is a doctor made a mistake and ended up being imprisoned. That . . . will have a chilling effect on their aggressiveness and efficiency" (Associated Press, 1995). According to the General Counsel of the Medical Society of the State of New York, the "prosecution of Dr. Einaugler has a chilling effect on the medical profession, but, moreover, has ominous implications for patients" (Moy, 1995).

Right after the decision in this case, the normally responsible *Wall Street Journal* published a hysterical op/ed piece that concluded ferociously:

The Einaugler verdict means that physicians are at the mercy and whim of any vindictive prosecutor trying to make a name for himself. The state will decide after the fact which clinical judgments are to be condoned or punished. The very basis of law, more important than justice or fairness, is expectability. A law may be stupid or cruel. But if you know in advance what's legal and what isn't, you can make a conscious decision about whether to cross the line. Doctors in New York no longer have that fundamental protection.

As unfair as the verdict is for physicians, its implications are more ominous for patients. Fear of malpractice suits already results in billions of dollars of unnecessary defensive medical tests and treatments. Watch those costs soar when the penalty for guessing wrong is a jail cell.

The verdict will force prudent doctors to be dangerously cautious. If deciding to monitor a patient rather than hospitalize him is criminal neglect, what doctor wouldn't call for the ambulance? The risks to the frail elderly of needless transfers shouldn't be underestimated. "Transfer trauma" is a real problem. But it may protect the physician who feels that a prosecutor might conclude—a few months later—that he was too slow to act. All patients should ask themselves: Can I rely on the advice of a doctor who's worried that his best judgment could result in his loss of liberty? (Crane, 1995)

These descriptions echo those of many other physicians. The general state of anxiety is made worse by the absence of any accepted national guidelines setting parameters to inform the exercise of presently unbridled prosecutorial discretion in the bringing of criminal charges against physicians related to end-of-life care (Lynn, 1994, p. 44).

It appears, thus, that medical practitioners and their advocates who support an interpretation of the Einaugler affair that "physicians who continue to hold to the tradition of putting the patient's interests first have little to fear from the criminal legal system, even as prosecutors in criminal cases begin to look more closely at the gross misconduct of physicians" (Allen, 1996) fall into a distinct minority. In addition to all the other factors influencing physician perceptions, the popular press reinforces a medical mind-set of apprehension toward the criminal justice system. The potential for misinformation and misunderstanding on the part of both physicians and the public is incalculable when, for instance, syndicated columnist Ann Landers (who is neither a physician, an attorney, nor a bioethicist) confidently but misleadingly advises a family upset at the physician's refusal to withdraw tube feeding from their elderly, emaciated, Parkinson's disease–ravaged relative: "The doctors' refusal to remove your mother-in-law's feeding tube was totally appropriate—not only from a medical viewpoint, but also legally. Had they removed the tube, they could have been charged with murder" (Landers, 1995). Headlines about other criminal prosecutions of physicians (Associated Press, 1996b), no matter how rare, reinforce the mind-set of apprehension.

As noted earlier in this chapter, physician anxiety about possible criminal prosecution also may encourage *under*aggressive care for dying patients, that is, failure to make beneficial treatments available. Physicians may feel inhibited from prescribing needed palliative care, specifically pain-reducing drugs, due to fear of running afoul of federal and state controlled-substances laws. Thus, the powerful specter of criminal prosecution, let alone potential conviction and punishment, may ethically skew treatment of the most vulnerable patient population in both overtreatment and undertreatment directions. In 1996 the Project on Legal Constraints on Access to Effective Pain Relief supported by the Mayday Fund and the Emily Davie and Joseph S. Kornfield Foundation unveiled model legislative proposals to address this situation.

Civil Litigation

A high percentage of physicians fear the possibility of being sued civilly for monetary damages for medical malpractice based on withholding or withdrawing life-sustaining medical interventions from critically ill and dying patients. This type of anxiety runs especially strong in the hospital setting, whose climate regarding medical decision making is often characterized by physicians through the use of such adjectives as "rights-centered," "adversarial," and "lawyerly" (Finucane, 1994). Too frequently, this means that "the legal, lawsuit environment and the regulatory environment, which were set up to protect patients, have the unintended side-effect of having a lot of people inappropriately treated" (Office of Technology Assessment, 1987, p. 311, quoted in Hill & Shirley, 1992, p. 23).

Physician fears of being sued by someone for something in these kinds of scenarios have been evident since Karen Quinlan's professional caregivers two decades ago cited apprehension of being sued for honoring, without prior judicial blessing, the Quinlan family's request to discontinue mechanical ventilation for their permanently vegetative daughter in the first American "right to die" case to become a judicial precedent (Meisel, 1996, p. 53; *In re Quinlan*, 1976). Because the *Quinlan* court was aware of this psychological cloud hanging over the physicians and the consequent anguish inflicted on the patient's family as a result of the physicians' fear of removing the ventilator, it took as its self-imposed duty to find "a way to free physicians, in the pursuit of their healing vocation, from possible contamination by self-interest or self-protection" (Rothman, 1991, p. 227). The approach of the New Jersey Supreme Court in *Quinlan*, as well as the U.S. Supreme Court's majority decision in *Cruzan* (1990), has been sternly criticized as an unwitting attack on both medical accountability and professionalism. According to Annas (1996), these and similar judicial rulings wrongly let physicians off the ethical hook upon which it is their proper role to squirm.

Nevertheless, and disturbingly, physician concern about the risk of being sued for malpractice in end-of-life undertreatment situations appears to have worsened over the years rather than abated (Goetzler & Moskowitz, 1991), despite the severe paucity of actual experience to support this consternation, and indeed despite a number of lawsuits filed against physicians for *over*treatment in these circumstances (Lewin, 1996). A 1995 government study confirmed that "concern over litigation may be an issue for both the facility and the direct provider. . . . Physicians may be apprehensive about being sued by a family member who wants a different level of care provided than specified in the patient's directive" (U.S. General Accounting Office, 1995, p. 16).

In his recounting of the *Kramp* case, attorney Fulton (1994, p. 583) repeatedly asked the hospital attorney who was cautioning the physicians against honoring the family's wishes to abate life-sustaining medical intervention precisely who he thought was likely to bring a malpractice lawsuit. The hospital counsel's reply, "Perhaps the parents, when they recover from their emotional turmoil, will feel guilty about the decision and sue the hospital," is either illogical or disingenuous in light of that same counsel's rejection of the parents' offer, through their attorney, to sign a hold harmless agreement.

Physician anxiety about family members as potential plaintiffs playing the litigation lottery at the professional's expense appears particularly sharp in cases of patients who are cognitively and / or emotionally incapable of making and expressing their own medical preferences (Schneiderman & Tertzel, 1995; Hanson, Danis, Mutran, & Keenan, 1994). The mysterious son or daughter from some distant place showing up uninvited and unexpected at the last minute to disrupt the harmonious caring scene with unreasonable demands for futile medical assaults on the patient they have previously neglected is a stereotype that intrudes into virtually every discussion of these questions (Lynn, 1994, p. 44; Molloy, Clarnette, Braun, Eisemann, & Sneiderman, 1991).

The aura of legal suspicion that may becloud the relationship between physicians and the families of critically ill and dying patients usually manifests itself in treatment being provided in accordance with the family member whose preferences may be interpreted as the most aggressive and interventionist. Put differently, the most affirmatively demanding relative wins; more is better when it comes to defensive medicine, here as elsewhere in the health care enterprise. This physician bias is exemplified in the sincere lament of one practitioner:

I have in my practice an individual who has cost approximately $2.5 million to maintain over the past six years. During the time I have followed her, she has not moved, spoken or given any indication of consciousness. She is being supported by a tube in her windpipe attached to a respirator, by a tube in her stomach to continuously feed her and by around-the-clock nursing care. . . . This is not the wish of her providers, who have repeatedly requested that she be allowed to die. The family has insisted that all of this be done, and in our present environment there is no good way to stop this futility. (Fowkes, 1994)

In other words, blind adherence to the wishes of perceived future plaintiffs is believed to pave the path of least resistance for the physician (Watts, 1992; Ely, Peters, Zweig, Elder, & Schneider, 1992; Kayser-Jones, 1990). Those caring for critically ill and dying patients ordinarily "cave in" to family demands because of a sincere (albeit almost always misplaced) fear of adverse legal consequences if they do not so comply. Taken to its illogical extreme, this fear results in such nonsensical behavior as asking families for their permission to remove respirators and feeding tubes from patients whose conditions satisfy the clinical and legal definition of brain death, as though there actually were a real choice to be made or any obligation to continue treating a corpse or any risk of liability for failing to do so. Excessive deference to families also causes damage in the realm of artificially created shortages of organs for transplantation, when families are permitted to refuse permission to remove organs from a recently deceased relative even when the deceased had left clear instructions—which ought to be legally binding—to remove and use those organs (Ladin, 1996; Spital, 1996).

Physicians in these circumstances also strive for family consensus, even or sometimes especially when there is a valid advance directive that flies in the face of family demands to "do everything," because physicians psychologically, not just legally, prefer to avoid interpersonal conflicts and confrontations whenever possible.

The problem often is that physicians hide behind their fear of malpractice any time an uncomfortable circumstance comes up. Doctors all make very bad lawyers, but that does not stop us from talking about it all the time. So doctors are always saying, I do not want to be sued, and beads of sweat are quite common. (Cassell, 1994, p. 43)

The ways in which physicians often use legal apprehensions as a pretext for engaging in conduct that is really driven wholly or partially by other forces, such as the physician's own psychological needs, are discussed in Chapter 2. In the end-of-life sphere, physicians' deviations from known patient wishes may also be blamed on legal apprehensions when they really stem more from communication difficulties, an ongoing ambivalence about power and control in the physician-patient relationship, and the defining of success in terms of bare life and death rather than meaningfulness to the patient (Gilligan & Raffin, 1996).

Physicians' felt legal need to appease family demands, even at the expense of ethical medical treatment of the patient, has been reinforced by a couple of relatively recent legal developments. These two developments, which most physicians interpret as making even more uncertain the liability climate confronting them in the end-of-life arena, are judicial decisions in so-called futility cases (Daar, 1995) and implementation of the Americans with Disabilities Act (ADA).

In the futility sphere, though there have been a few decisions of note (Miles, 1991), the Baby K case has received the most enormous attention in the popular and professional press. It involved an anencephalic infant whom physicians wanted to deny resuscitation attempts in the event of cardiac arrest because they felt that those attempts would provide no benefit, but whose mother insisted that resuscitation be attempted if the child were brought to the hospital's emergency room. The federal circuit court of appeals, in a decision that has drawn pointed legal derision (Annas, 1994), upheld the mother's right to insist that everything be done to keep the infant alive (*In the Matter of Baby K*, 1994). Many physicians have interpreted this decision expansively to compel legally the provision of as much medical intervention as any relative can think to demand. As one physician has written in exasperation, "Unless there is some legal relief from this condition, most physicians will probably continue to 'do everything' if the family so instructs, regardless of whether or not they feel it is in the patient's best interest" (Fronduti, 1994).

Congressional enactment of the ADA in 1990, 42 United States Code §12101–12213, has introduced another unknown legal variable into the equation. A number of physicians and other professionals express varying degrees of apprehension that the failure to be completely aggressive in providing life-sustaining medical interventions for every patient— regardless of the extent of their mental and/or physical disabilities— might expose the physician and others to civil damages in a lawsuit brought under the ADA, on the grounds of unlawful discrimination. Speculation on this point and on closely related issues has also begun to appear in the professional literature (Orentlicher, 1996).

Regulatory Sanctions

The negative influence of fear about legal repercussions on ethical practice may differ greatly depending on specific service delivery site. Anxiety about the imposition of regulatory sanctions, jeopardizing a facility's licensure status and certification for financially imperative Medicare and Medicaid participation, is especially powerful within heavily regulated nursing facilities. This mind-set frequently leads, in turn, to improper treatment of many nursing facility residents near the end of life.

In his thoughtful analysis of barriers to forgoing artificial nutrition and hydration in nursing facilities, legal scholar Alan Meisel (1995b) noted that "the myth persists among some—and perhaps many—nursing home personnel (probably reinforced by the practices of state Medicaid surveyors) that legal standards for dietary services mandate that nursing home residents who cannot be fed by mouth must have feeding tubes inserted and that anyone who has a feeding tube cannot have tube-feeding halted" (p. 380). According to Meisel, "The fundamental obstacle to enforcing the right to forgo artificial nutrition and hydration is not the law or its interpretation, but its incorrect application or the fear of its incorrect application by overzealous state regulators of long-term care facilities" (p. 379).

When objecting residents, families, or staff tacitly or explicitly call attention to the ethical dilemma created by harmful overtreatment, nursing facilities have an incentive to "turf" the difficult patient to other, more amenable providers (e.g., acute hospital, hospice, home) rather than risk the wrath of an upset surveyor. Such interinstitutional transfers are undertaken for the psychological benefit of the nursing facility, not its resident.

The possibility, however remote, of regulatory sanctions in the form of adverse state medical licensure actions such as suspension or revocation can also be an ominous influence of physician behavior. For instance, physicians who read in the American Medical Association's weekly newsletter (Associated Press, 1996c) about the travails of Dr. James Gallant, who had to defend himself against a complaint brought against him by the Oregon Board of Medical Examiners for ordering a muscle-relaxing drug that caused death for a suffering, brain-hemorrhaging seventy-eight-year-old patient at (he claimed) the behest of the patient and family, are not likely to be inspired to follow patient and family requests of this nature in their own future practices. Similarly, physicians who read Brian Bohlmann's (1997) description of his investigation by a state medical examining board (which totally exonerated him, by the way) because, he claims, of his attempts to make the family of a dying patient face the grim realities of their situation are likely to agree with Dr. Bohlmann's assessment that "withdrawing intensive care treatment in futile situations is not as simple as [an article author] imagines and may pose important [legal] risks to the treating physicians."

"WHAT JUST AIN'T SO"—SO WHAT?

An aphorism attributed to Will Rogers goes: "It ain't what people don't know that's so bad; it's what they know that just ain't so." Much of the legal anxiety influencing inappropriate medical treatment for critically ill and dying patients is fueled by misunderstanding and misinterpretation. For example, legal experts interviewed by the U.S. General Accounting Office indicated that when an individual's wishes are clear, difficulties in getting requests honored to withhold or withdraw artificial nutrition and hydration typically arise from confusion about the legal ramifications and not because there actually exists any legal impediment (U.S. General Accounting Office, 1995, p. 41). Writing about the psychological climate inspiring overtreatment, particularly unwanted tube feedings, in long-term care facilities, Meisel (1995b) has lamented:

> The commonly held myth that unless there is positive law—statute or regulation—that specifically states that something is permissible, it is impermissible. A corollary of this narrow view of law—probably held by many nonlawyers, but, incomprehensibly, by some lawyers too [see Chapter 4]—is that case law is not *real* law. . . . Those who operate nursing homes—and as difficult as it might seem, their lawyers too—either might not know about relevant case law within their own state or they might believe that such case law is not "really" law or is clearly subordinate to the statutes and regulations, rather than to be read *in pari materia* with them. (p. 380)

A thorough exegesis of right-to-die law is beyond the scope of this volume, and excellent accounts are available elsewhere (Meisel, 1995a; Keyes, 1995). In other venues, I have characterized the erroneous legal thinking surrounding this area as the myths of: simplicity (critical care decision making should be unambiguous and straightforward, and legal interference in medical affairs makes that process unnecessarily complex); intrusion; unreasonableness (because the law related to critical illness and dying is based solely on abstract theory and untouched by clinical realities, it is basically inconsistent with sound clinical judgment and ethical imperatives); inflexibility (legal requirements are too inflexible to accommodate clinical realities, the flip side of the myth that the law is too ambiguous to guide clinicians sufficiently); and lethargy (the claim that the law is too slow to respond to clinical controversies, which of course is the mirror image of the complaint that it is too anxious to intrude gratuitously into personal matters) (Kapp, 1986; Kapp & Lo, 1986).

According to calculations by the nation's leading authority on the legal aspects of dying (Meisel, 1996, pp. 68–69), somewhere between 0.2 and 0.5 percent of all American patient deaths since 1976 have been litigated in any manner, and between thirty-seven and fifty-five in ten million have been litigated to the point of yielding an appellate decision. These miniscule figures exist despite the fact that a high percentage of these patient deaths have involved conscious, purposeful decisions to withhold or withdraw some form(s) of life-prolonging medical intervention(s).

Nonetheless, however weak their factual foundations, the anxieties felt by physicians and other health care providers about potential criminal, civil, and/or regulatory liabilities are a real and palpable influence on the quality and humanity of medical care actually provided to the most vulnerable patients. This appears true even for physicians who intellectually understand that their own legal exposure is minimal; the very fact that their conduct in this most delicate of areas could conceivably be questioned in a legal context is enough to skew behavior erratically. Physician Jack McCue (1995) most assuredly is right when he urges, "The exaggerated fears of liability risks that pressure physicians and nurses to withhold palliative treatment or continue futile therapy in patients near the end of life must be addressed in a forthright fashion" (McCue, 1995, p. 1041). The American Geriatrics Society (Ethics Committee, 1995) has taken a formal position:

> Administrative and regulatory burdens that may serve as barriers to palliative care should be reduced. . . . Regulations intended to promote adequate nutrition for nursing home residents and laws intended to prevent assisted suicide and euthanasia should be written or revised so that these issues are not confused with proper palliative care decisions and treatment. (p. 578)

Thus, we see that, here as elsewhere within the physician-patient relationship, there is some tension between the physician's fear of undesired legal involvement, on one hand, and sound principles of medical ethics, on the other. Possible strategies for addressing, if not totally resolving, this tension are discussed in Chapter 7. First, though, we turn to the ways in which liability anxieties impinge on patients' prerogatives regarding everyday living (Chapter 5) and to the impact of managed care and a changing health care delivery and financing system on the ways in which physicians are likely to strike a balance between risk management and good medical ethics (Chapter 6).

NOTE

1. To its credit, the AHA was much more reasonable in the legal advice it provided in the subsequent, post-*Cruzan* (1990) version of these guidelines (American Heart Association, 1992, p. 2287).

REFERENCES

Allen, E. C. (1996). Doctors and the criminal law [Letter]. *New England Journal of Medicine, 334,* 196.

American Board of Internal Medicine. (1996a). *Caring for the dying: Identification and promotion of physician competency—educational resource document.* Philadelphia: ABIM.

American Board of Internal Medicine. (1996b). *Caring for the dying: Identification and promotion of physician competency—personal narratives.* Philadelphia: ABIM.

American Geriatrics Society Ethics Committee. (1995). The care of dying patients: A position statement. *Journal of the American Geriatrics Society, 43,* 577–578.

American Heart Association. (1992). Guidelines for cardiopulmonary resuscitation and emergency cardiac care. *Journal of the American Medical Association, 268,* 2171–2288.

Annas, G. J. (1996). Facilitating choice: Judging the physician's role in abortion and suicide. *Quinnipiac Health Law Journal, 1,* 93–112.

Annas, G. J. (1995). Medicine, death, and the criminal law. *New England Journal of Medicine, 333,* 527–530.

Annas, G. J. (1994). Asking the courts to set the standard of emergency care—the case of Baby K. *New England Journal of Medicine, 330,* 1542–1545.

Annas, G. (1978 February). The incompetent's right to die: The case of Joseph Saikewicz. *Hastings Center Report, 8*(1), 21–23.

Asch, D. A., Hansen-Flaschen, J., & Lanken, P. N. (1995). Decisions to limit or continue life-sustaining treatment by critical care physicians in the United States: Conflicts between physicians' practices and patients' wishes. *American Journal of Respiratory and Critical Care Medicine, 151,* 288–292.

Associated Press (1996a, September 16). Ethicist wants doctors to give more pain relief. *American Medical News, 39,* 26.

Associated Press (1996b, November 4). Physician charged with manslaughter after OR death. *American Medical News, 39,* 34.

Associated Press (1996c, August 5). Doctor accused of giving unwanted lethal injection. *American Medical News, 39,* 31.

Associated Press. (1995, March 17). Doctor will go to jail for fatality. *Dayton (OH) Daily News,* p. 3A.

Barber v. Superior Court. (1983). 147 Cal.App.3d 1006, 195 Cal. Rptr. 484.

Behr, D. J. (1994). Prescription drug control under the federal controlled substances act: A web of administrative, civil and criminal law controls. *Washington University Journal of Urban and Contemporary Law, 45,* 41–119.

Blum, R. H., Simpson, P. K., & Blum, D. S. (1990, September/October). Factors limiting the use of indicated opioid analgesics for cancer pain. *American Journal of Hospice & Palliative Care, 7,* 31–35.

Bohlmann, B. J. (1997). Letter. *Annals of Internal Medicine, 126,* 586.

Borneman, T., & Ferrell, B. R. (1996). Ethical issues in pain management. *Clinics in geriatric medicine, 12,* 615–628.

Brody, H. (1992). Assisted death—a compassionate response to a medical failure. *New England Journal of Medicine, 327,* 1384–1388.

Bruera, E., Fox, R., Chadwick, S., Brenneis, C., & MacDonald, N. (1987). Changing patterns in the treatment of pain and other symptoms in advanced cancer patients. *Journal of Pain & Symptom Management, 2*, 139–144.

Callahan, D. (1993). *The troubled dream of life.* New York: Simon & Schuster.

Cantor, N. L., & Thomas, G. C., III. (1996). Pain relief, acceleration of death, and criminal law. *Kennedy Institute of Ethics Journal, 6*, 107–127.

Caplan, A. L., Blank, R. H., & Merrick, J. C. (1992). *Compelled compassion: Government intervention in the treatment of critically ill newborns.* Totowa, NJ: Humana Press.

Cassel, C. K. (1994). Testimony. In U.S. Congress, Senate Committee on Finance. *Hearing: End of life issues and implementation of advance directives under health care reform.* 103rd Cong., 2nd Sess. Washington, DC: U.S. Government Printing Office.

Cassel, C. K., & Vladeck, B. C. (1996). ICD-9 code for palliative or terminal care. *New England Journal of Medicine, 335*, 1232–1233.

Cassell, E. (1994). Testimony. In U.S. Congress, Senate Committee on Finance. *Hearing: End of life issues and implementation of advance directives under health care reform.* 103rd Cong., 2nd Sess. Washington, DC: U.S. Government Printing Office.

Cassell, E. (1991). Relief of suffering: The doctor's mandate. *Journal of Palliative Care, 7*, 3–4.

Casswell, D. G. (1990). Rejecting criminal liability for life-shortening palliative care. *Journal of Contemporary Health Law and Policy, 6*, 127–144.

Clark, F. I. (1996). Making sense of *State v. Messenger. Pediatrics, 97*, 579–583.

Cleland, C. S. (1987). Barriers to the management of cancer pain. *Oncology, 1* (Supp. 2), 19–26.

Commonwealth v. Kominsky. (1976). 361 A.2d 794 (Sup.Ct. Pa.).

Commonwealth v. Youngkin. (1981). 427 A.2d 1356 (Sup.Ct. Pa.).

Crane, M. (1995, February 21). Practice medicine, land in jail. *Wall Street Journal,* p. A24.

Crowley, P. C. (1994). No pain, no gain? The Agency for Health Care Policy & Research's attempt to change inefficient health care practice of withholding medications from patients in pain. *Journal of Contemporary Health Law and Policy, 10*, 383–403.

Cruzan v. Director, Missouri Department of Health. (1990). 497 U.S. 261.

Cummins, R. O. (1992). Matters of life and death: Conversations among patients, families, and their physicians. *Journal of General Internal Medicine, 7*, 563–565.

Daar, J. F. (1995). Medical futility and implications for physician autonomy. *American Journal of Law & Medicine, 21*, 221–240.

Danis, M., Southerland, L. I., Garrett, J. M., Smith, J. L., Hielema, F., Pickard, C. G., et al. (1991). A prospective study of advance care directives for life-sustaining care. *New England Journal of Medicine, 324*, 882–887.

Desbiens, N. A., Wu, A. W., Broste, S. K., Wenger, N. S., Connors, A. F., Jr., Lynn, J., et al. (1996). Pain and satisfaction with pain control in seriously ill hospitalized adults: Findings from the SUPPORT research investigations. *Critical Care Medicine, 24*, 1953–1961.

Dubler, N. N. (1993). Balancing life and death—proceed with caution. *American Journal of Public Health, 83*, 23–25.

Dull, S. M., Graves, J. R., Larsen, M. P., & Cummins, R. O. (1994). Expected death and unwanted resuscitation in the prehospital setting. *Annals of Emergency Medicine, 23*, 997–1002.

Ely, J. W., Peters, P. G., Zweig, S., Elder, N., & Schneider, F. D. (1992). The physician's decision to use tube feedings: The role of the family, the living will, and the *Cruzan* decision. *Journal of the American Geriatrics Society, 40*, 471–475.

Emanuel, L. (1993, Spring). Advance directives: What have we learned so far? *Journal of Clinical Ethics, 4*(1), 8–16.

Ferrell, B. R., McCaffery, M., & Rhiner, M. (1992). Pain and addiction: An urgent need for change in nursing education. *Journal of Pain & Symptom Management, 7*, 117–124.

Fins, J. J. (1996). Physician-assisted suicide and the right to care. *Cancer Control, 3*, 272–278.

Finucane, T. E. (1994). Inside the Commission. *Bifocal* (Newsletter of the ABA Commission on Legal Problems of the Elderly), *15*(3), 11.

Finucane, T. E. (1993). Legislating care for her mother. *American Journal of Medicine, 95*, 658–659.

Fowkes, B. (1994, September 19). The right to die [Letter]. *Newsweek*, p. 16.

Fried, T. R., Stein, M. D., O'Sullivan, P. S., Brock, D. W., & Novack, D. H. (1993). Limits of patient autonomy: Physician attitudes and practices regarding life-sustaining treatments and euthanasia. *Archives of Internal Medicine, 153*, 722–728.

Fronduti, R. A. (1994). Do everything [Letter]. *Annals of Internal Medicine, 121*, 900.

Fulton, G. B. (1994). The "non-declarant" in a PVS: Adventures in Ohio's legal wonderland. *Ohio Northern Law Review, 20*, 571–595.

Gauthier, C. C. (1993). Philosophical foundations of respect for autonomy. *Kennedy Institute of Ethics Journal, 3*, 21–37.

Gianelli, D. M. (1996a, September 23/30). Treat pain, avert suicide. *American Medical News, 39* (1), 27.

Gianelli, D. M. (1996b, November 11). Medical boards, legislatures expand view of pain control. *American Medical News, 39* (1), 38–39.

Gillick, M. R. (1994). *Choosing Medical Care in Old Age.* Cambridge, MA: Harvard University Press.

Gilligan, T., & Raffin, T. A. (1996). Whose death is it, anyway? *Annals of Internal Medicine, 125*, 137–141.

Goetzler, R. M., & Moskowitz, M. A. (1991). Changes in physician attitudes toward limiting care of critically ill patients. *Archives of Internal Medicine, 151*, 1537–1540.

Green v. Abrams (1993). 984 F.2d 41 (2 Cir.).

Griffin, E. A. (1997). Letter. *Annals of Internal Medicine, 126*, 587.

Gupta, K. L. (1991). CPR in nursing home patients: British and American approaches [Letter]. *Journal of the American Geriatrics Society, 39*, 1241–1244.

Hanson, L. C., Danis, M., Mutran, E., & Keenan, N. L. (1994). Impact of patient incompetence on decisions to use or withhold life-sustaining treatment. *American Journal of Medicine, 97*, 235–241.

Hansot, E. (1996). A letter from a patient's daughter. *Annals of Internal Medicine, 125,* 149–151.

Harvard Law Review Staff (1990). Developments in the law: Medical technology and the law. *Harvard Law Review, 103,* 1519–1676.

Hastings Center (1987). *Guidelines on the termination of life-sustaining treatment and the care of the dying.* Briarcliff Manor, NY: Hastings Center.

Hill, T. P., & Shirley, D. (1992). *A good death: Taking more control at the end of your life.* Reading, MA: Addison-Wesley Publishing Company.

Hodges, M. O., & Tolle, S. W. (1994). Tube-feeding decisions in the elderly. *Clinics in Geriatric Medicine, 10,* 475–488.

Hodges, M. O., Tolle, S. W., Stocking, C., & Cassel, C. K. (1994). Tube feeding: Internists' attitudes regarding ethical obligations. *Archives of Internal Medicine, 154,* 1013–1020.

Hoffmann, D. E., Zimmerman, S. I., & Tompkins, C. J. (1996). The dangers of directives or the false security of forms. *Journal of Law, Medicine & Ethics, 24,* 5–17.

In the Matter of Baby K. (1994). 16 F.3d 590 (4th Cir.).

In re Quinlan. (1976). 70 N.J. 10, 355 A.2d 647, *cert. denied,* 429 U.S. 922.

Jacobson, J. A., Kasworm, E., Battin, M. P., Francis, L. P., Green, D., Botkin, J., et al. (1996). Advance directives in Utah: Information from death certificates and informants. *Archives of Internal Medicine, 156,* 1862–1868.

Joint Commission on Accreditation of Healthcare Organizations (1996). *Accreditation manual for hospitals.* Chicago: JCAHO.

Kapp, M. B. (1996). Therapeutic jurisprudence and end-of-life medical care: physician perceptions of a statute's impact. *Medicine and Law, 15,* pp. 201–217.

Kapp, M. B. (1995a). Problems and protocols for dying at home in a high-tech environment. In J. D. Arras (Ed.), *Bringing the hospital home: Ethical and social implications of high-tech home care,* pp. 180–196. Baltimore: Johns Hopkins University Press.

Kapp, M.B. (1995b). Medical decisionmaking for older adults in institutional settings: Is beneficence dead in an age of risk management? *Issues in Law & Medicine, 11,* 29–46.

Kapp, M. B. (1994). Futile medical treatment: A review of the ethical arguments and legal holdings. *Journal of General Internal Medicine, 9,* 170–177.

Kapp, M. B. (1992). State statutes limiting advance directives: Death warrants or life sentences? *Journal of the American Geriatrics Society, 40,* 722–726.

Kapp, M. B. (1986). Decision-making in critical care: Is the law an impediment or a scapegoat? *Critical Care Medicine, 14,* 247–250.

Kapp, M. B., & Lo, B. (1986). Medical decision making for the demented and dying. *Milbank Quarterly, 64* (Supplement 2), 163–202.

Kayser-Jones, J. (1990). The use of nasogastric feeding tubes in nursing homes: Patient, family, and health care provider perspectives. *Gerontologist, 30,* 469–479.

Kayser-Jones, J., & Kapp, M. B. (1989). Advocacy for the mentally disabled elderly: A case study analysis. *American Journal of Law & Medicine, 14,* 353–376.

Keyes, W. N. (1995). *Life, Death, and the Law: A Sourcebook on Autonomy and Responsibility in Medical Ethics (2 volumes)*. Springfield, IL: Charles C. Thomas, Publisher.

Ladin, L. (1996, March 14). Death and the maiden. *Wall Street Journal*, p. A14.

Landers, A. (1995, November 19). Reader pleads for elimination of feeding tube. *Dayton Daily News*, p. 5E.

Lasch, K., & Carr, D. B. (1996). Pain assessment in seriously ill patients: Its importance and need for technical improvement. *Critical Care Medicine, 24*, 1943–1944.

Lewin, T. (1996, June 2). Suits accuse medical community of ignoring "right to die" orders. *New York Times*, pp. A1, 28–29.

Lo, B., & Steinbrook, R. (1991). Beyond the *Cruzan* case: The U.S. Supreme Court and medical practice. *Annals of Internal Medicine, 114*, 895–901.

Lo., B., Saika, G., Strull, W., Thomas, E., & Showstack, J. (1985). Do not resuscitate decisions: A prospective study at three teaching hospitals. *Archives of Internal Medicine, 145*, 1115–1117.

Longergan, T. (1996, October 21). Predatory prosecutions regarding pain treatments put physicians at risk [Letter]. *American Medical News, 39*, 19.

Lynn, J. (1996). Caring at the end of our lives. *New England Journal of Medicine, 335*, 201–202.

Lynn, J. (1994). Testimony. In U.S. Congress, Senate Committee on Finance. *Hearing: End of life issues and implementation of advance directives under health care reform*. 103rd Cong., 2nd Sess. Washington, DC: U.S. Government Printing Office.

Macklin, R. (1993). *Enemies of patients: How doctors are losing their power and patients are losing their rights*. New York: Oxford University Press.

Major, D. (1986). The medical procedures for providing food and water: Indications and effects. In J. Lynn (Ed.), *By no extraordinary means: The choice to forgo life-sustaining food and water*. Bloomington, IN: Indiana University Press.

McClung, J. A., & Kramer, R. S. (1990). Legislating ethics: Implications of New York's do-not-resuscitate law. *New England Journal of Medicine, 323*, 270–272.

McCrary, S. V., Swanson, J. W., Perkins, H. S., & Winslade, W. J. (1992). Treatment decisions for terminally ill patients: Physicians' legal defensiveness and knowledge of medical law. *Law, Medicine & Health Care, 20*(4), 364–376.

McCue, J. D. (1995). The naturalness of dying. *Journal of the American Medical Association, 273*, 1039–1043.

McIntyre, K. M. (1983). Medicolegal aspects of cardiopulmonary resuscitation (CPR) and emergency cardiac care (EEC). In K. M. McIntyre and A. J. Lewis (Eds.), *Textbook of Advanced Cardiac Life Support*, pp. 275–291. Dallas: American Heart Association.

Meisel, A. (1996). The "right to die": A case study in American lawmaking. *European Journal of Health Law, 3*, 49–74.

Meisel, A. (1995a). *The right to die*, 2nd ed. (2 volumes). Colorado Springs, CO: Wiley Law Publications.

Meisel, A. (1995b). Barriers to forgoing nutrition and hydration in nursing homes. *American Journal of Law and Medicine, 21*, 335–381.

Meisel, A. (1992). The legal consensus about forgoing life-sustaining treatment: Its status and its prospects. *Kennedy Institute of Ethics Journal, 3*, 309–345.

Miles, S. H. (1991). Informed demand for "non-beneficial" medical treatment. *New England Journal of Medicine, 325*, 512–515.

Miller, D. K., Coe, R. M., & Hyers, T. M. (1992). Achieving consensus on withdrawing or withholding care for critically ill patients. *Journal of General Internal Medicine, 7*, 475–480.

Molloy, D. W., Clarnette, R. M., Braun, E. A., Eisemann, M. R., & Sneiderman, B. (1991). Decision making in the incompetent elderly: The daughter from California syndrome. *Journal of the American Geriatrics Society, 39*, 396–399.

Mondragon, D. (1987). U.S. physicians' perceptions of malpractice liability factors in aggressive treatment of dying patients. *Medicine & Law, 6*, 441–447.

Moskop, J. C., & Saldanha, R. L. (1986, April). The Baby Doe rule: Still a threat. *Hastings Center Report, 16*, 8–14.

Moskowitz, E. H., & Nelson, J. L. (1995, November–December). Dying well in the hospital: The lessons of SUPPORT. *Hastings Center Report, 25* (Special Supplement), S1–S36.

Moss, R. J., & LaPuma, J. (1991, January–February). The ethics of mechanical restraints. *Hastings Center Report, 21*, 22–25.

Moy, D. R. (1995, March 13). The doctor as criminal [Letter]. *Wall Street Journal*, p. A15.

Murphy, D. J., Murray, A. M., Robinson, B. E., & Campion, E. W. (1989). Outcomes of cardiopulmonary resuscitation in the elderly. *Annals of Internal Medicine, 111*, 199–205.

Murray, T. H. (1985, June). The final, anticlimactic rule on Baby Doe. *Hastings Center Report, 15*, 5–9.

Nelson, L. J., & Cranford, R. E. (1989). Legal advice, moral paralysis and the death of Samuel Linares. *Law, Medicine & Health Care, 17*, 316–324.

Nuland, S. B. (1994). *How we die: Reflections on life's final chapter.* New York: Alfred A. Knopf.

Office of Technology Assessment, U.S. Congress. (1987). *Life-sustaining technologies and the elderly.* Washington, DC: U.S. Government Printing Office.

Orentlicher, D. (1996). Destructuring disability: Rationing of health care and unfair discrimination against the sick. *Harvard Civil Rights–Civil Liberties Law Review, 31*, 49–87.

Page, L. (1996, July 22). Model law sought to protect prescribing for intractable pain. *American Medical News, 39*, 25.

Parker, L. S., & Buller, T. G. (1994, July–August). Case study: A hard policy to swallow. *Hastings Center Report, 24*(4), 23–24.

Payne, K., Taylor, R. M., Stocking, C., & Sachs, G. A. (1996). Physicians' attitudes about the care of patients in the persistent vegetative state: A national survey. *Annals of Internal Medicine, 125*, 104–110.

People v. Anyakora (1993). 162 Misc.2d 47, 616 N.Y.S.2d 149 (Sup.Ct.).

People v. Cabral. (1983). 141 Cal.App.3d 148, 190 Cal.Rptr. 194 (Ct.App. 2 Dist.).

People v. Coe. (1988). 71 N.Y.2d 852, 527 N.Y.S.2d 741, 522 N.E.2d 1039 (Ct.App.).

People v. Einaugler. (1994). 618 N.Y.S.2d 414 (App.Div.2d Dept.).

People v. Ketchum. (1974). 361 N.Y.S.2d 911 (Ct.App.).

People v. Protopappas. (1988). 246 Cal. Rptr. 915 (Cal.App.4 Dist.).

Pollack, S. (1996). Detours on the road to autonomy: A critique of the New York State do-not-resuscitate law. *Archives of Internal Medicine, 156,* 1369–1371.

Post, S. G., & Whitehouse, P. J. (1995). Fairhill guidelines on ethics of the care of people with Alzheimer's disease: A clinical summary. *Journal of the American Geriatrics Society, 43,* 1423–1429.

President's Commission for the Study of Ethical Problems in Medicine and Biomedical and Behavioral Research (1982). *The ethical and legal implications of informed consent in the patient-practitioner relationship.* Washington, DC: U.S. Government Printing Office.

Protecting patients in pain [Editorial]. (1996, September 9). *American Medical News, 39,* 23.

Quill, T. E. (1995). "You promised me I wouldn't die like this!" A bad death as a medical emergency. *Archives of Internal Medicine, 155,* 1250–1254.

Quill, T. E. (1994). Risk taking by physicians in legally gray areas. *Albany Law Review, 57,* 693–708.

Quill, T. E. (1993). The ambiguity of clinical intentions. *New England Journal of Medicine, 329,* 1039–1040.

Quill, T. E. (1992). Letter. *New England Journal of Medicine, 326,* 495.

Rhymes, J. A. (1996). Barriers to effective palliative care of terminal patients. *Clinics in Geriatric Medicine, 12,* 407–416.

Rothman, D. J. (1991). *Strangers at the bedside: A history of how law and bioethics transformed medical decision making.* New York: Basic Books.

Rouse, F. (1994). Decision making about medical innovation: The role of the advocate. *Albany Law Review, 57,* 607–616.

Sachs, G. A., & Siegler, M. (1991). Guidelines for decision making when the patient is incompetent. *Journal of Critical Illness, 6,* 348–359.

Sachs, G. A., Miles, S. H., & Levin, R. A. (1991). Limiting resuscitations: Emerging policies in the emergency medical system. *Annals of Internal Medicine, 114,* 151–154.

Schneiderman, L. J. (1994). Medical futility and aging: Ethical implications. *Generations, 18*(4), 61–65.

Schneiderman, L. J., & Teetzel, H. (1995). Who decides who decides? When disagreement occurs between the physician and the patient's appointed proxy about the patient's decision-making capacity. *Archives of Internal Medicine, 155,* 793–796.

Schneiderman, L. J., & Jecker, N. S. (1995). *Wrong medicine: Doctors, patients, and futile treatment.* Baltimore: Johns Hopkins University Press.

Schneiderman, L. J., Kronick, R., Kaplan, R. M., Anderson, J. P., & Langer, R. D. (1992). Effects of offering advance directives on medical treatment and costs. *Annals of Internal Medicine, 117,* 599–606.

Shapiro, R. S. (1994a). Liability issues in the management of pain. *Journal of Pain & Symptom Management, 9,* 146–152.

Shapiro, R. S. (1994b). Legal bases for the control of analgesic drugs. *Journal of Pain & Symptom Management, 9,* 153–159.

Skelly, F. J. (1994a, March 7). Painful truth. *American Medical News, 37,* 17.

Skelly, F. J. (1994b, May 9). Painful barriers. *American Medical News, 37,* 15.

Skelly, F. J. (1994c, May 16). Price of pain control. *American Medical News, 37,* 13–15.

Skelly, F. J. (1994d, August 15). Fear of sanctions limits prescribing of pain drugs. *American Medical News, 37,* 13.

Smith, A. M. (1995). Criminal or merely human? The prosecution of negligent doctors. *Journal of Contemporary Health Law and Policy, 12,* 131–153.

Smith, G. P., II (1996). *Legal and healthcare ethics for the elderly.* Washington, DC: Taylor & Francis.

Snider, G. L. (1995). Withholding and withdrawing life-sustaining therapy: All systems are not yet "go." *American Journal of Respiratory Critical Care Medicine, 151,* 279–281.

Solomon, M. Z., O'Donnell, L., Jennings, B., Guilfoy, V., Wolf, S. M., Nolan, K., et al. (1993). Decisions near the end of life: Professional views on life-sustaining treatments. *American Journal of Public Health, 83,* 14–23.

Spital, A. (1996). Mandated choice for organ donation: Time to give it a try. *Annals of Internal Medicine, 125,* 66–69.

State v. Brenner. (1986). 486 So.2d 101 (La.).

State v. Killory. (1976). 243 N.W.2d 475 (Wisc.).

State *v. Serebin.* (1984). 350 N.W.2d 65 (Wisc.).

State v. Warden. (1991). 813 P.2d 1146 (Utah).

SUPPORT Principal Investigators (1995). A controlled trial to improve care for seriously ill hospitalized patients. *Journal of the American Medical Association, 274,* 1591–1598.

Symposium. (1996). Physician-assisted suicide. *Duquesne Law Review, 35,* 1–532.

Teno, J., Lynn, J., & Phillips, R. S. (1994). Do formal advance directives affect resuscitation decisions and use of resources for seriously ill patients? *Journal of Clinical Ethics, 5,* 28–30.

Tonelli, M. R. (1996). Pulling the plug on living wills: A critical analysis of advance directives. *Chest, 110,* 816–822.

U.S. General Accounting Office. (1995). *Patient Self-Determination Act: Providers offer information on advance directives but effectiveness uncertain.* GAO/HEHS-95-135. Washington, DC.

van der Poel, C. J. (1996, May/June). Ethical aspects of palliative care. *American Journal of Hospice and Palliative Care, 13,* 49–55.

Van Grunsven, P. R. (1996). Criminal prosecution of health care providers for clinical mistakes and fatal errors: Is "bad medicine" a crime? *Journal of Health and Hospital Law, 29,* 107–120.

Wanzer, S. H., Adelstein, S. J., Cranford, R. E., Federman, D. D., Hook, E. D., Moertel, C. G., et al. (1984). The physician's responsibility toward hopelessly ill patients. *New England Journal of Medicine, 310,* 955–959.

Watts, D. T. (1992). The family's will or the living will: Patient self-determination in doubt. *Journal of the American Geriatrics Society, 40,* 533–534.

Wolf, A. M. D., & Becker, D. M. (1996). Cancer screening and informed patient discussions: Truth and consequences. *Archives of Internal Medicine, 156,* 1069–1072.

Wynia, M. K. (1994). Do everything [Letter]. *Annals of Internal Medicine, 121,* 900–901.

Young, E. W. D., & Stevenson, D. K. (1990). Limiting treatment for extremely premature, low-birth-weight infants. *American Journal of Diseases of Children, 144,* 549–552.

Zinberg, J. M. (1989). Decisions for the dying: An empirical study of physicians' responses to advance directives. *Vermont Law Review, 13,* 445–491.

5

Who Is Responsible for This? Everyday Patient Intrusions to Protect the Provider

For the most part, this book examines the influence of legal anxieties on the ethical conduct of health care providers, primarily physicians, within the context of "medical" matters. These "medical" matters have been defined thus far in rather traditional terms, to include such scientific and/or empirical activities as diagnostic tests and procedures, drug prescription, and therapeutic interventions initiated on the basis of a physician's order and carried out under a physician's supervision and pertaining directly to the patient's bodily health.

The ethical lobotomizing of the health professions resulting from their pervasive obsession with liability risks is by no means limited in its impact to "medical" matters so narrowly defined. The health care delivery system wields an enormous power over the everyday lives of individuals in ways that extend well beyond the diagnosis and treatment of strictly medical maladies.

For example, in 1994 Drake Center in Cincinnati, a long-term care facility, cruelly refused fifty-three-year-old Barry Belinky's request to stay overnight in the bed of his wife of thirty-one years (Barisic, 1996). Diane Belinky, age 54, was paralyzed and barely able to speak because of a brain aneurysm rupture two years earlier, and the attending physicians held out no hope of recovery or improvement. This refusal of the husband's overnight stay request was issued, according to a memo written by Drake's vice-president of nursing, because the facility feared being sued (by whom, for what damages, and with what likelihood of success were items not specified by that v.p.) in the event sexual relations between this middle-aged chemist and his retired synagogue administrator wife were to occur.

Human tragedies bordering on farces of this nature are not isolated incidents. This chapter aims to broaden our thinking about the concept of defensive medicine by examining how the paternalistic behavior undertaken by health care providers in the name of regrettable but necessary risk management frequently creates ethical damage in its wake. It does this by significantly limiting patient prerogatives in such areas as physical and chemical restraints, assisted living, selecting and directing home- and community-based services, guardianship, and involuntary civil commitment and third-party warnings of danger. It is driven mightily by providers' apprehension of being accosted by the accusation "Who is responsible for this?" whenever there is an adverse outcome. On the part of health care professionals, too frequently there is palpable apprehension, in the cynical but not unfounded spirit of no good deed going unpunished, of being held accountable for respecting and abetting ill-fated patient and/or family choices by an after-the-fact jury of lawyers, regulators, funders, and the press and public. It is an illustration of our modern "catastrophobia" or "episodic panic," a state of mind that elevates the avoidance of the horrible into the equivalent of achieving good. In sports terms, it is playing the game not to win but to keep from losing.

RESTRAINTS

At least until the past decade, the use of physical devices and prescribed drugs for their effect as patient restraints was quite commonplace in hospitals and nursing facilities (as well as within psychiatric institutions). Even today, the prevalence of restraint use in health care settings within the United States—an intervention that legally requires a specific physician's explicit order—substantially exceeds that found in otherwise comparable settings elsewhere in the industrialized world. To a significant extent, this situation represents another example of inappropriately defensive conduct based on a highly questionable interpretation of legal dangers. Here, as elsewhere in this book, overblown apprehension of theoretical litigation and liability possibilities induces clinical practice that violates important ethical principles while, paradoxically, increasing more than diminishing the providers' actual legal exposure.

Nursing Facilities

In this country, the historical use of restraints in nursing facilities at much higher rates than those reported elsewhere in the world has taken place despite substantial evidence of restraints' deleterious effects on the residents' physical and mental well-being (Evans & Strumpf, 1989). Overuse of restraints, that is, their initial and continued invocation in circumstances where less-restrictive or -intrusive alternatives are reasonably available to accomplish the legitimate goal of resident safety and/or the safety of others, violates the individual's interests in autonomy (self-determination), beneficence (doing good), and nonmaleficence (Primum non nocere, "First, do no harm").

However, many long-term care administrators and their medical and nursing staffs have overridden resident and family (Kanski, Janelli, Jones, & Kennedy, 1996) objections, or else accede automatically to uninformed family requests for the use of restraints, without exploring less-intrusive alternatives. This represents, at least in part, a provider response to anxiety about liability exposure connected to resident injuries associated with falls or wandering. Provider practice that has encompassed routine, indiscriminate utilization of restraints, without meaningful exploration of less-restrictive alternatives, has at best misperceived the realistic relative legal risks involved. This misperception and related practice unfortunately are often the result of hysterical, unreflective risk management advice proffered to the long-term care industry (see Chapter 3) (Kapp, 1994a).

Research, as opposed to the mythology and gossip that sometimes infiltrate the health care delivery environment, reveals that far more lawsuits have been filed based on injuries occasioned by the inappropriate application of restraints than based on wrongful failure to apply restraints (Johnson, 1990; Kapp, 1992). The numbers of cases in both categories are relatively small. Although even less common, criminal charges against long-term care corporations and specific staff members have been prosecuted on theories of negligent homicide for the deaths of residents by vest strangulation. In some states (e.g., California), the inappropriate use of physical restraints is classified as a form of criminal elder abuse.

Even if a civil lawsuit based on failure to restrain were filed, available defenses would include compliance with standards of care based on evidence rather than custom (Rubenstein, Miller, Postel, & Evans, 1983) and the resident's or family's informed, voluntary assumption of risk. Present government regulations, particularly federal Medicare/Medicaid standards promulgated at 45 Code of Federal Regulations §483.13 to implement the Nursing Home Quality Reform Act (part of the Omnibus Budget Reconciliation Act [OBRA] of 1987) and FDA standards implementing the Safe Medical Devices Act, Public Law No. 101-629, also contain presumptions against the use of restraints. The burden rests with the provider to demonstrate the appropriateness of restraints in terms of needed (no reasonable alternative) protection (beneficence and nonmaleficence) for the particular resident during the specific time period.

Thus, a realistic perspective on relative risks would favor a presumption against the routine use of restraints. The ethical principles of resident autonomy and beneficence point in the same direction (Moss & LaPuma, 1991; Strumpf & Evans, 1991).

Furthermore, financial considerations are in agreement with this approach. The nursing facility industry complained bitterly, upon enactment of the 1987 Nursing Home Quality Reform Act, that reduced reliance on the use of restraints would necessarily increase staffing requirements and hence inflate the cost of care. The recent experience of the many facilities that have moved successfully toward restraint-free or restraint-reduced environments has been overwhelmingly the opposite. These providers have found that fewer restraints lead to a less agitated resident population that can be managed well with fewer, not more, nursing staff. Moreover, the time that staff would otherwise spend on the imposition, monitoring, and correction of restraints is eliminated (Phillips, Hawes, & Fries, 1993).

Hospitals

The use of restraints, particularly physical devices or materials that mechanically restrict the patient's freedom of movement, physical activity, or normal access to his or her body, also has been widespread over the years in American hospitals. They have been employed in general medical and surgical units, in emergency and psychiatry departments, and in critical care settings.

The clinical and legal implications of using restraints in the hospital environment have been largely overlooked until quite recently. Today, though, these implications are the subject of increasingly intense scrutiny by health professionals, regulators, patient advocates, and commentators (Reigle, 1996). (Eventually, similar concerns will also be analyzed in the context of restraint use in home care [Kapp, 1995a]). This scrutiny must entail a critical examination of the usually erroneous but nonetheless widely shared clinical and legal presumptions that have tended to guide the behaviors of hospital medical and nursing staffs in this arena (Matthiesen, Lamb, McCann, Hollinger-Smith, & Walton, 1996).

Most often, health professionals attempt to justify their use of restraints as a matter of patient protection, especially the prevention of serious injury falls that might expose the hospital as well as individual professionals to lawsuits and legal liability (Francis, 1989). However, the evidence that restraints accomplish this objective—that is, that they actually prevent serious fall injuries or that removing them contributes to an increase in such injuries—is somewhere between scant and non-existent (Capezuti, Evans, Strumpf, & Maislin, 1996). At the same time, the significant injury risks in *using* restraints are substantial and well-documented (Miles & Meyers, 1994; Robinson, Sucholeiki, and Schocken, 1993; Miles & Irvine, 1992).

Thus, in acute care settings as in long-term care, most health care professionals and administrators have mistakenly overestimated the therapeutic and prophylactic value of restraints for patients and underestimated their dangers in terms of causing patient injuries. Consequently, those individuals most responsible for making and carrying out decisions regarding restraint practice also have erroneously presumed that their liberal use constitutes good risk management.

In fact, in hospitals as in nursing facilities, the overuse of physical restraints is self-defeating as a defensive strategy. Many nosocomial and iatrogenic injuries actually are the result of reliance on restraints. It thus stands to reason that cases holding providers liable in the absence of restraints have been far outweighed, in both number and size, by legal judgments awarded and settlements negotiated on the basis of inappropriate ordering of restraints, failure to monitor and correct their harmful effects on the patient, or errors in the way that the restraint was mechanically applied. Claims have been filed both on theories of negligence (an unintentional or accidental deviation below acceptable professional standards) and battery (intentional, unconsented-to, offensive invasion of the patient's bodily integrity).

Relevant regulatory requirements push in the same restraint reduction direction as does the weight of malpractice case precedent. For instance, hospitals that operate nursing facility units or "swing beds" must act in compliance with the restraint limitation sections of the Nursing Home Quality Reform Act and its implementing regulations.

Furthermore, in the last half decade the federal Food and Drug Administration (FDA) has turned its attention to the status of physical restraints as medical devices. The FDA has issued a medical bulletin entitled "Potential Hazards With Protective Restraint Devices" as a Safety Alert to hospital administrators, nursing directors, and directors of emergency room services. Since 1992, restraints must be labeled as "prescription-only" devices. Beginning in 1996, restraining devices require FDA prior approval for marketing and sale.

Perhaps most importantly, the FDA actively maintains complaint files concerning such devices. The information contained in those files is accessible by members of the public, including plaintiffs' attorneys, upon request under the federal Freedom of Information Act (FOIA), 5 United States Code §552. Under the Safe Medical Devices Act (SMDA) passed in 1990 and alluded to in the previous discussion about nursing facilities, hospitals and other health care facilities are obliged to report incidents connecting a medical device and a patient's death to the FDA on Form 3500A within ten working days. If earlier problems involved in the use of specific devices have been made a matter of public record and a hospital nonetheless condones the use of those devices by its staff on its patients, and injuries then occur for which the patient or her representative seeks financial compensation, the hospital's defense usually will be a difficult one. It will have the burden of persuading the trier-of-fact (ordinarily a jury in medical malpractice litigation) that restraint use was appropriate in the particular situation even in the face of information the hospital had or should have had about the hazards associated with the device.

Pertinent standards of the Joint Commission on Accreditation of Healthcare Organizations (JCAHO) are a quasi-regulatory force in restraint reduction for the 90-plus percent of hospitals that apply for JCAHO accreditation. In 1996, JCAHO published a new chapter of its standards (Standard TX) for hospitals that deals exclusively and very specifically with the use of physical restraints and seclusion. The stated goal of this new standard is unequivocally to "create a physical, social, and cultural environment limiting restraint and seclusion use to clinically appropriate and adequately justified situations or that actually reduces its [sic] use through preventive or alternative strategies."

In Chapter 2, I discuss the concept of fear of legal consequences being used as a pretext to mask other motivations for certain conduct. The overuse of restraints offends ethical sensibilities most of all when it is fueled not by a sincere but misguided concern about risk management but by the citation (consciously or subconsciously) of a legally defensive rationale as only a pretext for furthering the interests of underlying professional bias and administrative convenience. Especially where the autonomy and well-being of patients and families are at stake, health professionals have an ethical responsibility to guard against attempts to justify conduct that in fact is driven by unexamined professional prejudices about patient care or explicit or implicit administrative policies grounded on management rather than patient interests. The ethical integrity of health care providers demands that their ultimate product be good decisions and actions, not excuses.

ASSISTED LIVING

Assisted living is a rapidly emerging, albeit inexactly defined, mode of combining housing with limited health and social services for persons—primarily but not necessarily the elderly—who are impaired in the performance of certain activities and instrumental activities of daily living (ADLs and IADLs), but who do not require care at the level of a skilled-nursing facility. Many individuals could benefit from this relatively new type of residential arrangement, some for lengthy periods of their lives (Wilson, 1996; Kane & Wilson, 1993).

But essential to the success of this developing service model is intellectual and emotional commitment by service providers and families to the underlying philosophical paradigm of homelike individual autonomy and self-determination, rather than the traditional institutional care watchwords of safety and protection at all costs. Under the newer approach, the vast majority of assisted living consumers are presumed to be adults who are capable of formulating, expressing, and acting upon their own values and preferences regarding both major life decisions and smaller, but nevertheless exquisitely important, choices arising in everyday life. Adding vigor to this paradigm is widespread recognition that in the past protective provider conduct justified under the traditional protective paradigm often had proceeded beyond beneficence to programs of intrusive and restrictive forms of paternalism.

There are a variety of impediments, however, to translation of this paradigm shift from theoretical acceptance to tangible, operational reality. Among the most powerful of these inhibiting forces is the ubiquitous anxiety about exposure to potential litigation and legal liability that health and human service professionals mentally associate with the service provision environment generally, and specifically with permitting and even facilitating patients/clients to make and implement autonomous "bad" choices that place themselves at risk of avoidable injury.

These law-related apprehensions not infrequently have influenced provider behavior in a paternalistic direction, powered by the assumption that restricting consumer control over living arrangements and service provision details thereby increases the level of safety surrounding the consumer's setting. Thus, the intimidating malpractice and regulatory climate provides a great temptation to restrict self-determination by dictating to assisted living consumers such particulars of their lives as meal content, bath schedules, medication timing, whether the favorite throw rug may remain on the living room floor, and the like.

If the assisted living movement is to fulfill its potential on behalf of individuals who desire and need such a residential option, it will be essential to harness much of the law-related anxiety that now stands as a barrier to the fundamental paradigm shift from imposed protection to meaningful consumer participation in planning and decision making. Legal risks must be put into some realistic perspective, and effective risk management strategies must be identified. Special attention needs to be given to strategies founded on a process of negotiated or managed risk that incorporates communication conducted and agreements reached among provider, consumer, and—as necessary and appropriate—family members or others who are acting on the consumer's behalf (Kapp & Wilson, 1995).

CONSUMER DIRECTED HOME- AND COMMUNITY-BASED CARE

Even with the apparent collapse, at least for the time being, of initiatives for major overhaul of the total American health care delivery and financing system, there remains a good deal of public discussion about the need for a more rational, comprehensive system of long-term care (LTC) in this country. Current debate about this topic offers the opportunity to move from the traditional model basically of professional dominance, in which the individual has only the right of negative autonomy to accept or reject recommended interventions, more toward a right of positive autonomy (Collopy, 1990) encompassing proactive participation in the actual design and implementation of personal service plans (Kapp, 1996).

Various possible models for financing and delivering home- and community-based LTC services ought to be evaluated according to their likelihood of promoting important policy goals. The precept of personal autonomy has emerged in recent discussions and consumer polls (U.S. General Accounting Office, 1994, p. 15) as a fundamental value to be preserved and enhanced in any expanded program of home- and community-based LTC. This precept is embodied in some form in virtually all client Bill of Rights statements regarding home care (e.g., National Council on Aging, 1988).

There is a growing body of empirical evidence that the perception of personal control plays a critical role in an individual's long-run physical and emotional health and well-being (Rodin, 1986). There are strong arguments that enhanced consumer autonomy is associated with the practical benefits of fostering independence over time, reducing the person's risk of abuse and neglect by others, and increasing satisfaction with those aspects of service that consumers feel are important indicators of quality of care. Feelings of control contribute to positive behaviors, tending to reduce the phenomenon of "learned helplessness" (Avorn & Langer, 1982).

Especially in the home- and community-based context, individual control concerning the routine and minutiae of care may be central. For instance, what time will the personal assistant or home health aide arrive? What food will be brought into the home, how will it be prepared, and when will it be served? When will the individual get dressed, and with what attire? When will various activities be scheduled? What will be cleaned in the home, and when? How will furniture be arranged? Most important, how will the personal assistant or home health aide be located, hired, and fired (Ferrara, 1990, pp. 427–430)?

Despite what we know about the importance of personal control over these and similar issues, several significant obstacles discourage home- and community-based LTC from actually becoming more consumer autonomy–friendly in practice. One problem is our obsession with formal structures for accountability. The last decade has produced a remarkable evolution (bordering on revolution) in public attitudes regarding the wisdom and efficacy of government oversight, through extensive command-and-control regulation, of the conduct of programs designed to improve the public's well-being. Earlier, the prevailing wisdom favored detailed, comprehensive regulation concerning all aspects of a public program's design and operation as the only means to assure satisfactory quality for the consumer and accountability for the taxpayer. Today, by contrast, a significant consensus has coalesced around the position that intrusive regulation often acts less as an accountability tool than as an inflexible barrier to appropriate consumer choice and professional discretion, making programs less rather than more responsive to intended beneficiaries. The rallying cry today is that "regulation is currently part of the problem" when it comes to promoting consumer autonomy (Hofland & David, 1990, p. 93).

Another obstacle to consumer autonomy at present is the proclivity of case managers, other gatekeepers, and direct service providers to focus on the person's professionally perceived service needs and risks of harm. This emphasis on expertly determined needs (prevalent even in supposed "client oriented" models of case management [U.S. General Accounting Office, 1993, p. 14]) and risks is driven largely by the ethical principle of beneficence that underlies the philosophy, education, and practice of the helping professions. It is underscored by the predilection of many managers and professionals to assume too readily decisional incapacity and dependence on the part of their consumers.

Some individuals, particularly the elderly and disabled, certainly face the possibility of neglect or abuse if left on their own. The problem is that, taken too far, professional behavior driven by the desire to help and protect vulnerable consumers (and, not incidentally, by the desire to avoid legal accusations of substandard professional performance) can diverge widely from the consumer's own goals of choice and satisfaction, reinforce learned helplessness, and amount to parentalism rather than support (Kane, 1988).

Some providers resist consumer control over the details of a service plan because they interpret this movement as decreasing the caregivers' control over prevention or mitigation of risk factors. Control, even over consumer objection, ordinarily is asserted in the name of beneficence. Justice Brandeis warned Americans three-quarters of a century ago, in his dissenting opinion in *Olmstead v. United States*, 277 U.S. 438, 479 (1928), that "experience should teach us to be most on our guard to protect liberty when the Government's purposes are beneficent."

The same admonition might be applied to many health and human service agencies. Besides its adverse implications for autonomy, over-protectionism at its extremes can lead to professional conduct that really is counterproductive and even harmful to consumer welfare (for example, regulations that do not permit an individual's dedicated, willing, and otherwise able family members to perform certain in-home tasks because they lack formal professional credentials) and that there-fore also effectively violates the precepts of beneficence and non-maleficence (Mahowald, 1993; Powderly, 1993).

The philosophically and educationally based managerial profes-sional bias in favor of externally imposed protection of the consumer from any foreseeable harm frequently is seriously exacerbated by anx-iety on the part of gatekeepers and service providers about potential exposure to civil liability for negligence (i.e., malpractice) if the foreseen risk materializes and the consumer suffers an injury. Certainly, a move-ment toward greater use of consumer- and family-directed home- and community-based care entails real legal implications, relating both to possible claims of professional malpractice (Kapp, 1995b) and to ques-tions of regulatory, employment, tax, and workers' benefits liability (e.g., income tax reporting, payment of Social Security, unemployment insurance, workers' compensation) (Sabatino & Litvak, 1995). Concerns by gatekeepers and service providers about their legal risks in these emerging scenarios are widespread and sincere, and they exert a robust influence over professional behavior.

Actual legal risks and responsibilities arising in this sphere should be addressed through targeted, coherent risk management efforts (Kapp, 1995b) and, where necessary, public policy changes or clarifications (Kapp, 1996). However, in this area as elsewhere, many of the popularly held and repeated perceptions of legal risk are quite free-floating and exaggerated. These sorts of professional biases and anxieties must be addressed head-on and ideally replaced by a recognition that many consumers of home- and community-based services and their families are quite willing to accept responsibility for the risks and consequences of their care decisions. Such acceptance of responsibility, as well as the willingness of service professionals to accept that acceptance, is essential to achieving real consumer autonomy and choice about important matters in this setting. As one noted gerontologist wrote about his own feelings as he steadily declined in his own home:

> Be my friend, for I need one, but do not become my manager. And remember me, as my life and identity erode, as a person, not a case.
> Let me live and grow old in a place I know. It is enough that my body becomes a stranger and my thoughts unclear.
> Somewhere in here is still the aspiring hopeful person you once said would inherit the future. (Ossofsky, 1993)

The ethical significance of the desired paradigm shift in health services delivery from an external, policing model to a more internal, client-centered one was described eloquently by one philosopher:

> The responsibility to make and live with one's own choices lies at the heart of true autonomy. What makes persons morally special —and what renders them worthy of respect—is their capacity to be held morally accountable for the choices they make and for the kinds of people they become through their exercise of self-determination. They, unlike non-autonomous creatures, can be expected to justify their actions and are subjected to praise, blame, and other characteristically moral appraisals. Freedom is an important prerequisite of responsibility, because we cannot be accountable for that which we cannot freely control. But responsibility, rather than freedom, is the moral heart and soul of autonomy. (Morreim, 1994, p. 97)

UNNECESSARY AND PREMATURE GUARDIANSHIPS[1]

There are an increasing number of people—primarily but not exclusively the elderly—today with some degree of mental impairment in their ability to engage in rational decision-making processes and to reach and communicate autonomous, authentic choices concerning financial and personal (including medical) matters. Social strategies are necessary to protect persons from harm without excessively intruding on their autonomy, once they have been assessed as having impaired decisional capacity.

Some persons with impaired capacity are subjected to formal guardianship or conservatorship proceedings (Kapp, 1994b). A judicial official declares the person (the ward) legally incompetent and appoints someone else as the guardian or conservator with legal authority to make decisions on behalf of the ward. Sometimes there is no meaningful choice about this course of action, because less-intrusive alternatives have been tried and have failed—for example, when a party in a position of trust has abused or exploited the impaired person.

A number of policy considerations, however, argue against overuse of this formal legal mechanism. Guardianships frequently are expensive, time-consuming, and emotionally tumultuous; they may result in unnecessary deprivation of basic civil liberties. Yet, in many cases, they provide the ward with little meaningful protection against abuse and exploitation (American Bar Association, 1989).

Anxieties about their own potential exposure to litigation and legal liability on the part of health and social service professionals frequently leads to defensive practice with negative ethical connotations in at least two guardianship-related senses. First, legal fears may unduly skew physicians' assessments of their patients' decisional capacity in a manner that contributes to the filing of and/or supports guardianship petitions that might have been avoided. Second, legal as well as other forces act as impediments to the creation and continued operation of programs and services that could delay or even obviate the need for many guardianships.

Skewing Capacity Assessments

Especially for older patients being treated in institutional settings, physicians' legal risk aversion often leads to a bias toward reliance (frequently overreliance) on surrogates—particularly family members with or without explicit legal authority—to make decisions. Sometimes this practice substitutes for a careful assessment of the patient's own functional capacity to engage in a rational decision-making process regarding the specific issue to be decided. In many situations (see Chapter 4), physicians and other health care providers ordinarily have a greater anxiety about a patient's relatives as potential malpractice plaintiffs than they do about the patient herself taking on that role. Thus, it is not uncommon for deference to family demands in many cases to trump patient involvement where there is any question raised about the patient's decision-making capacity. This may be true even when the professional team suspects or believes that the family is acting contrary to the patient's best interests (Kayser-Jones & Kapp, 1989).

As discussed in Chapter 2, health care providers sometimes cite liability fears as a pretext for rationalizing conduct that actually is driven more by professional prejudice (e.g., old, frail nursing home patients obviously are unable to make their own decisions, or else they would be young, healthy, and attending professional conferences) or administrative convenience. This type of rationalization may be conscious or subconscious. It undeniably is considerably more efficient to deal with an articulate relative than to do a thorough evaluation on an impaired person, to tailor specific decision-making processes to the patient's specific capabilities, to help the patient to maximize limited but real capabilities, and to document all of these efforts. Nonetheless, this is not a categoric description of provider behavior. In many instances, liability fears are sincerely felt by providers who believe that their options for delivering quality care that respects the patient's autonomy and dignity are unduly constrained.

Although in theory decision-making capacity is just as essential for a patient to give valid informed consent to a recommended medical or social intervention as to withhold such consent and object to the professional's proposal, relatively rarely is careful attention actually paid to assessing the capacity of nonobjecting patients. This is particularly true if surrogate decision makers are available and everyone is in agreement on the desired course of action. Because the professional's anxiety usually focuses on the family as potential plaintiff, a cooperative family allays the professional's worries and quenches the thirst for further reflection on the patient's capacity.

Sometimes there is a question about patient decision-making capacity, and no suitable surrogate is reasonably available or there is disagreement (among rival surrogates, between surrogate and patient, or between surrogate and provider) that is not resolved through an informal communication and negotiation process. In such circumstances, professionals may be fearful of liability for proceeding on the sole basis of the patient's own express wishes (assuming the patient can even express wishes). In these circumstances, the professional may insist—in the name of risk management—on judicial appointment of a formal substitute decision maker. This approach is contrary to the "least restrictive alternative" position that most cases involving decision making for persons of questionable functional status are better dealt with outside of the court system (Schmidt, 1995; Annas & Densberger, 1984).

Nevertheless, in situations in which the informal process of communication and negotiation will not work, the judicial forum indeed may be a less restrictive alternative than abandoning the questionably competent patient's well-being to an absence of advocacy and oversight. It is not the ultimate resort to the courts that is per se objectionable, but rather a practice of automatic reliance on the pacifying protection of a judicial decree instead of first exploring available nonjudicial options for safeguarding both the patient and provider.

In nursing homes, an especially unfortunate variation of this dynamic sometimes take place (Kapp, 1990). Because the available pool of potential guardians often is especially shallow in that setting, an undue preoccupation with liability may result in defaulting decisions to a crisis mode. The *de facto* but not *de jure* (not formally adjudicated) decisionally incapacitated patient may be transferred to a hospital where medical intervention occurs on the basis of the emergency exception to the ordinary informed consent rule. The ability to shift the most difficult decisional capacity cases to other providers—hospitals, hospices, and in extreme cases mental institutions—is a fundamental but disquieting characteristic of contemporary nursing home care.

It should also be acknowledged that physician behavior in assessing the capacity of patients in both institutional and community settings is influenced by the reimbursement practices of third-party payers in compensating physicians for rendering cognitive services. This economic disincentive to devote effort toward finding and cultivating decisional capacity in borderline situations reinforces the negative impact of legal apprehension (see Chapter 6).

Alternatives to Guardianship

In developing alternatives to guardianship, society must balance the ethical principles of self-determination, on one hand, and nonmaleficence and beneficence, on the other. Optimal methods will minimize external intrusion into the individual's freedom and autonomy, while safeguarding her from potential harms of impaired personal and financial decision making.

Much recent attention has been paid to exploring and developing viable alternatives to plenary (complete) guardianship of indefinite duration that strike an acceptable balance between protection and independence (Stiegel, 1992). However, substantial anecdotal evidence suggests a serious impediment to the development and implementation of such guardianship alternatives, namely, anxiety concerning potential exposure to legal liability in the event of harm to the questionably capable person (Kapp, 1995c).

More specifically, some factors encourage unduly conservative behavior in pursuing alternative-to-guardianship activities. Others discourage professionals, volunteers, and proprietary and community agencies from undertaking activities that might reduce, divert, prevent, or delay the need for formal guardianships. The principal barriers are (a) fear of lawsuits brought by consumers or their family members against the service provider, and (b) difficulty in obtaining and/or affording professional liability insurance to indemnify and defend professionals, volunteers, and agencies in the event of a lawsuit questioning the appropriateness of their activities undertaken to forestall or eliminate the need for formal guardianship.

I use the phrase "alternative-to-guardianship services" (AGSs) here to represent a host of legal tools, social services, benefit programs, and residential options that enhance or maintain a cognitively or emotionally impaired person's individual autonomy. These approaches share a common goal: to delay or avoid the deprivation of civil rights and liberties, loss of control, and financial and emotional costs associated with formal plenary guardianship. An AGS also may divert from the guardianship system persons who do not meet the applicable legal criteria for guardianship but who might be at risk of guardianship imposition anyway if not assisted with certain aspects of everyday living. Examples of AGSs are case management services, adult protective services, and daily money management and representative payee services.

Fear of legal liability in the event of client harm inhibits the development and expansion of AGSs and may exert a negative effect on guardianship services themselves. Nearly all service providers (or would-be service providers) experience some degree of anxiety concerning possible legal liability. In a survey I conducted in 1991–92 (Kapp, 1995c), a typical comment was that of the director of a midwestern statewide alliance on aging, who said that service providers in his state are "paranoid about liability. . . . In any type of service delivery, the second word out of everyone's mouth is, 'Can I get sued?'" An executive director of a senior citizen center in a western state expanded on this sentiment when explaining that there are two main hurdles to overcome in aging services: funding and liability.

A heightened level of fear of liability can result when a neighboring service provider is sued or threatened with a lawsuit. This was the case for the money management community in northern California in the aftermath of the disintegration of a well-known and highly respected organization in the San Francisco area, Support Services for Elders, due to massive embezzlement by a trusted, long-standing employee.

However, in most cases fear of liability appears to be generic and free-floating in nature. When pressed, service providers had difficulty articulating specific worries. Few were able to cite an actual case upon which they based their fears, and even fewer had been sued or personally involved in defending a legal action. According to one public guardian, "Confusion is running so high that we can't even talk about liability concerns. It is an unintelligent fear that is a cover for lack of available interventions and knowledge . . . . A general attitude exists that if we notice liability concerns, then our liability will increase."

Meeting a dependent, impaired person's needs often may be a very complex and challenging task. A care manager described feeling as if her job were full of "mini-minefields." Approaches to cases vary, even within the best social service system. The depth and quality of family involvement may affect choices made regarding treatment plans and care options. Different practitioners may approach a case in different ways, thus resulting in potentially internally inconsistent practices within an agency. Services, treatment philosophies, and areas of expertise also vary from agency to agency.

In certain instances, issues may become convoluted as the interests of family members and the consumer come into conflict. For example, such a problem might occur when a family caregiver who has lived with a person faces the prospect of selling that person's home to pay for medical or long-term-care expenses. It may be in the best interest of the consumer to have the home sold, but such a sale would also deprive the family member of a home.

Providers, too, can feel trapped in conflicts involving the balancing of autonomy and beneficence (Kane & Caplan, 1993). If, for example, an elderly person living alone begins to have difficulty remembering to shut off the stove, the agency may fear liability for the benevolent and protective act of unplugging the stove because the person may fall and injure himself while trying to plug it in again. Yet, on the other hand, a service provider deciding to take a stance that protects the consumer's autonomy may fear liability for nonfeasance if it does nothing and the home burns down the next time that the man forgets to turn off the stove. Worse yet would be the neighbor's home burning down too.

Anxiety about liability can come from many sources, some of which go beyond the realm of legal requirements and insurance-dictated practices. A majority of individuals interviewed for my earlier study stated that the general litigious nature of today's society, plus heightened media coverage of isolated exorbitant damage awards or sensationalized accounts of alleged cases of abuse and neglect or other malpractice by service providers, strongly influence their perceptions about potential legal liability. For some in the field, the mere prospect of facing the time, cost, and bad publicity associated with defending against a lawsuit (even and perhaps especially a nuisance claim) was cited as nearly as inhibiting as the prospect of an actual judgment of liability and awarding of damages.

Agencies interviewed for the earlier study who were or could have been providing AGSs indicated fairly easy access to legal advice and commented that such access has both a positive and negative impact on the provider's attitude concerning legal liability risks. A "go ahead and let them sue" mentality exists among a few providers having ready

access to legal resources, particularly when legal defense is at no charge to the provider. Overall, attorneys appear to be not only helpful in solving legal issues pertaining to AGSs but equally adept at pointing those issues out—thus both inflaming and mitigating the service provider's level of liability anxiety.

Providers pointed out that increasing caseloads, declining funds, and reduced staffing play important roles in increasing anxiety about liability for them. Caseworkers, supervisors, and administrators are aware that decreasing personal contact with consumers is an inevitable by-product of an ever-increasing client caseload. This factor, when coupled with an undertrained and overworked staff, may create a high-risk situation ripe for staff's making mistakes or missing important details.

Liability perceptions also seem to hinge on the degree to which industry standards have been developed, although such standards may have opposing effects. First, industry standards provide a "roadmap" for service providers to follow in many common situations (see discussion of clinical practice parameters in Chapter 8). This gives the provider generalized guidelines that may help to reduce liability anxiety. At the same time, however, strong industry standards also help define a legally objective measure against which the reasonableness of the service provider's conduct may be judged. This is felt to improve a plaintiff's chance to prove substandard care when the provider has deviated from the agreed-upon measure, an essential element of any successful malpractice lawsuit.

Because many AGSs comprise a new and growing enterprise, service providers often are still unable to take advantage of established industry standards, ethical guidelines, or professional practice parameters that might assist them in determining reasonable, appropriate behavior. There is a lag in the broad-based acceptance and implementation of industry standards for AGS services. Few providers now understand that compliance with industry standards can supply a powerful defense to a claim of malpractice.

Another key liability anxiety factor appears to be what the provider personally has at stake. This might include the provider's reputation, business, personal assets, or career goals. The opportunity to obtain or afford adequate insurance coverage may mitigate financial concerns related to defending against many types of potential lawsuits. However, insurance coverage does not necessarily rid the provider of anxiety surrounding the possible loss of reputation or stymied career progress that may accompany charges of alleged wrongdoing.

The owner of a private case management service, whose business had been in existence for nearly a decade, summed it up: "My fear is very real. My partners and I not only risk potentially losing our company, but our personal assets as well." Although the owners had run an ethical business for years, the interviewee described the terrifying thought that it could be destroyed almost overnight if the media obtained, augmented, and sensationalized claims of damaging or embarrassing activity. The owners would be left to deal with the aftermath of the negative press coverage and public impressions that would inevitably follow even a frivolous claim.

Finally, two interviewees believed that capable, autonomous, and informed consumers are better able to recognize substandard care or individual rights violations and therefore may pose a greater risk of suing a service provider than their more severely cognitively impaired peers. Likewise, family members, friends, or an outside advocacy network may assist in bringing legal action against service providers that abuse or exploit a consumer. At least in some instances, it appears that consumer and family education and empowerment, though playing a crucial ethical role in protecting the vulnerable, may heighten provider liability anxiety by extending the provider's potential risk of exposure to legal action.

A significant number of individuals and agencies interviewed for the AGS study perceived court-approved transactions to be preferable to alternative substitute decision-making arrangements not falling under direct court supervision. Many service providers consider formal court arrangements such as guardianship to be safer than alternative service arrangements, particularly in high-risk situations. After handling a number of cases dealing with family infighting and potential abuse, one typical case manager concluded that her preference is always for court-appointed surrogates, instead of less-intrusive alternatives like powers of attorney. This prevalent attitude creates serious implications for the autonomy of persons who are not capable of total independence, although some might argue that autonomy is most fully protected against abuse and exploitation under the procedural due process model of formal guardianship.

Some service professionals who were serving as either limited or plenary guardians for clients cited uneasiness over ambiguities in state guardianship statutes. Providers also wondered about liability associated with failure to adequately perform a statutory requirement (for example, a social worker's removing a ward from a dangerous living situation prior to obtaining, as required by state statute, court approval to change the ward's residence). Other service providers acting as financial and medical surrogate decision makers worried about liability issues that could emerge around the meaning of general statutory requirements, such as acting like a "prudent person" or in the "best interest" of the ward.

Perceived fear of liability not only impedes AGS providers and sponsors but also deters other parties from acting on or honoring alternatives to guardianship. Many physicians, health care facilities, and financial institutions are hesitant, or even refuse, to honor validly drafted durable power of attorney instruments. This behavior is partly due to confusion surrounding the legal and practical ramifications of this evolving form of decision-making mechanism, especially in light of ambiguous state statutes. Government agencies such as the Department of Veterans Affairs (VA) and the Social Security Administration (SSA) also generally refuse to honor privately executed powers of attorney, insisting instead on representative payee appointments or pushing for guardianship declarations.

Interviewees for the AGS study suggested that third-party recalcitrance in honoring guardianship alternatives may serve as a smokescreen covering for other underlying problems, rather than resting on the pure liability concerns that many third parties profess. For example, some banks may be reluctant to invest the time required to determine the validity of an AGS arrangement. The time, staff, and expertise required to check the documents can translate into additional costs for both the third party and the service providers, thus making it attractive to follow the "safer" route of honoring only standardized documents (i.e., documents written by that particular third party itself) or formally sanctioned court relationships such as guardianships.

In sum, providers of AGSs, as well as the liability insurance industry, exhibit a pervasive, though largely uninformed, anxiety regarding the threat of potential liability for services delivered to nonindependent consumers. Actual and imagined laws, voluntary professional standards, and customs have combined to inhibit many health and social service professionals, potential volunteers, governing boards, administrators of proprietary and community agencies, and insurance companies from performing or insuring activities designed to meet the needs of cognitively or emotionally impaired persons without formal plenary guardianship.

The accuracy of service provider and insurer perceptions is almost immaterial. Liability anxiety has already infiltrated service providers' business practices and has stymied providers' interaction with consumers and family members. Despite the lack of actual litigation in this sphere, many vulnerable individuals and families are turned away because they are seen as possible legal threats to the service provider. Crucially needed services such as money management and transportation, as well as the volunteer components of some programs, are hardest hit by service providers who decide to mitigate potential losses by avoiding, eliminating, or limiting certain types of "riskier" areas of service delivery.

INVOLUNTARY COMMITMENT AND WARNING THIRD PARTIES

Every state has enacted statutes that permit the involuntary (civil) commitment to a state owned or licensed mental health institution of individuals who are mentally ill and seriously, imminently dangerous to themselves or to others. Involuntary confinement based on danger to self is an exercise of the state's inherent *parens patriae* power to protect those who cannot adequately care for themselves, and commitment predicated on danger to others represents the state's police power to protect and promote the general health, safety, welfare, and morals of the community (Appelbaum, 1994, pp.17–70).

Involuntary commitments ordinarily are based on a designated tribunal finding the necessary elements of mental illness and danger by at least clear and convincing evidence (*Addington v. Texas*, 441 U.S. 418 [1979]). Ordinarily, the expert opinion and recommendation of one or more psychiatrists form the central basis for initiation of a commitment petition and for the commitment verdict. These opinions and recommendations involve predictions of future danger if involuntary confinement is not imposed on the proposed mental patient.

The ability of psychiatrists to make such professional predictions accurately and dependably enough to justify depriving individuals of their freedom by holding them against their wishes in public mental institutions has long been a subject of heated controversy among mental health and legal practitioners and researchers (Monahan & Steadman, 1994). Some psychiatrists indicate a propensity among many of their colleagues to initiate and support involuntary commitment petitions in dubious circumstances, due to apprehension of adverse legal consequences in the event commitment is not sought and actual harm to or by the patient materializes. Put differently, psychiatrists may err on the side of involuntary commitment when they fear being sued by someone acting on behalf of the injured patient or injured third party for letting the sick, violent patient go free; even when unsure, many psychiatrists are tempted to be influenced by the perception that the legal risks associated with false positives (unnecessarily restricting the patient's freedom) are not nearly as great as those associated with false negatives (not confining the truly dangerous). Even if the tribunal ultimately dismisses the commitment petition and releases the individual, or the individual converts to voluntary admission status before the hearing is conducted, most psychiatrists feel more protected legally by virtue of having argued in favor of commitment (Brown & Rayne, 1989; Lidz, Mulvey, Appelbaum, & Cleveland, 1989; Appelbaum, 1984).

A related manifestation of liability anxiety–inspired behavior of primary relevance to mental health professionals concerns warning third parties of potential dangers posed by mentally ill patients residing in the community. A series of judicial decisions and state statutes emerging over the past two decades has established in most jurisdictions a legal duty on the part of mental health professionals to give notice to third parties of dangers of harm posed to them by a professional's patient (Appelbaum, 1994, pp. 71–113). The precise contours and extent of this duty vary significantly among jurisdictions.

Psychiatrists uniformly claim that they and their peers, well aware of and driven (Schopp, 1991) by knowledge of the legal duty to warn and fear of potential liability for violating that responsibility, are much more likely to issue third-party warnings regarding their patients than they otherwise would be. This tendency to warn is manifested not only in gray areas but even in many cases where the mental health professional firmly believes that the danger has very little chance of really materializing. Again, the substantial and immediate danger of harming the patient through false or unnecessary third-party warnings usually is given less weight than the much more speculative risk of negative legal consequences for the professional based on the remote possibility that the patient will harm a third party in a manner that should have been anticipated and prevented by the professional.

Anxiety about potential liability to injured third parties may affect in myriad other ways the conduct of physicians besides those practicing psychiatry. For instance, primary care physicians and neurologists may collaborate with family members of early stage Alzheimer's disease victims to restrict a patient's driving opportunities prematurely out of excessive concern about lawsuits brought by strangers who might be injured in a car accident with the patient (Post & Whitehouse, 1995, p. 1424).

CONCLUSION

In this chapter, I have examined several selected areas within which a perceived tension between patient autonomy, on one hand, and safety (physical for the patient and legal for the provider), on the other hand, usually encourages health care professionals to impinge upon patient prerogatives and freedoms in often mundane but important ways (Collopy, 1995). Whereas those who attempt to deny altogether the existence of this tension (Raymond & Wentworth, 1993) may be acting more than a bit naively, matters often are unnecessarily exacerbated by exaggerated perceptions and misrepresentations of the legal risks involved. To the extent that those risks can be placed in a more realistic perspective, along with the implementation of other strategies discussed in this chapter and in Chapter 7, valuable inroads may be made in untying the hands of both professionals (figuratively) and patients (sometimes literally).

NOTE

1. This section of Chapter 5 is based in part on work conducted under sponsorship of the Retirement Research Foundation.

REFERENCES

Addington v. Texas, 441 U.S. 418 (1979).

American Bar Association, Commission on the Mentally Disabled and Commission on Legal Problems of the Elderly. (1989). *Guardianship: An agenda for reform*. Washington, DC: ABA.

Annas, G. J., & Densberger, J. (1984). Competence to refuse medical treatment: Autonomy versus paternalism. *University of Toledo Law Review, 15*, 561–596.

Appelbaum, P. S. (1994). *Almost a revolution: Mental health law and the limits of change*. New York: Oxford University Press.

Appelbaum, P. S. (1984). Hospitalization of the dangerous patient: Legal pressures and clinical responses. *Bulletin of the American Academy of Psychiatry and the Law, 12*, 323–329.

Avorn, J., & Langer, E. (1982). Induced disability in nursing home patients: A controlled trial. *Journal of the American Geriatrics Society, 30*, 397–400.

Barisic, S. (1996, February 23). Man sues to stay with wife. *Dayton Daily News*, p. 4B.

Brown, J., & Rayne, J. T. (1989). Some ethical considerations in defensive psychiatry: A case study. *American Journal of Orthopsychiatry, 59*, 534–541.

Capeziut, E., Evans, L., Strumpf, N., & Maislin, G. (1996). Physical restraint use and falls in nursing home residents. *Journal of the American Geriatrics Society, 44*, 627–633.

Collopy, B. J. (1995). Safety and independence: Rethinking some basic concepts in long-term care. In L. B. McCullough and N. L. Wilson (Eds.), *Long-term care decisions: Ethical and conceptual dimensions*, pp. 137–152. Baltimore: Johns Hopkins University Press.

Collopy, B. J. (1990). Ethical dimensions of autonomy in long-term care. *Generations, 19* (Supp.), 9–12.

Evans, L. K., & Strumpf, N. E. (1989). Tying down the elderly: A review of the literature on physical restraint. *Journal of the American Geriatrics Society, 37*, 65–74.

Ferrara, P. J. (1990). Expanding autonomy of the elderly in home health programs. *New England Law Review, 25,* 421–455.

Francis, J. (1989). Using restraints in the elderly because of litigation. *New England Journal of Medicine, 320,* 870–871.

Hofland, B. F., & David, D. (1990). Autonomy and long-term-care practice: Conclusions and next steps. *Generations, 14* (Supp.), 91–94.

Johnson, S. H. (1990). The fear of liability and the use of restraints in nursing homes. *Law, Medicine & Health Care, 18,* 263–273.

Kane, R. A. (1988). Case management: Ethical pitfalls on the road to high-quality managed care. *Quality Review Bulletin, 14,* 161–166.

Kane, R. A. & Caplan, A. L. (Eds.). (1993). *Ethical conflicts in the management of home care: The case manager's dilemma.* New York: Springer Publishing Company.

Kane, R. A., & Wilson, K. B. (1993). *Assisted living in the United States: A new paradigm for residential care for frail older persons.* Washington, DC: American Association of Retired Persons.

Kanski, G., Janelli, L., Jones, H., & Kennedy, M. (1996). Family reactions to restraints in an acute care setting. *Journal of Gerontological Nursing, 22*(6), 17–22.

Kapp, M. B. (1996). Enhancing autonomy and choice in selecting and directing long-term care services. *Elder Law Journal, 4,* 55–97.

Kapp, M. B. (1995a). Restraining impaired elders in the home environment: Legal, practical, and policy implications. *Journal of Case Management, 4,* 54–59.

Kapp, M. B. (1995b). Family caregiving for older persons in the home: Medical-legal implications. *Journal of Legal Medicine, 16,* 1–31.

Kapp, M. B. (1995c). Alternatives to guardianship: Enhanced autonomy for diminished capacity. In M. Smyer, K. W. Schaie, and M. B. Kapp (Eds.), *Older Adults' Decision-Making and the Law,* pp. 182–201. New York: Springer Publishing Company.

Kapp, M. B. (1994a). Physical restraints in hospitals: risk management's reduction role. *Journal of Healthcare Risk Management, 14,* 3–8.

Kapp, M. B. (1994b). Ethical aspects of guardianship. *Clinics in Geriatric Medicine, 10,* 501–512.

Kapp, M. B. (1992). Nursing home restraints and legal liability: Merging the standard of care and industry practice. *Journal of Legal Medicine, 13,* 1–32.

Kapp, M. B. (1990). Liability issues and assessment of decision-making capability in nursing home patients. *American Journal of Medicine, 89,* 639–642.

Kapp, M. B., & Wilson, K. B. (1995). Assisted living and negotiated risk: Reconciling protection and autonomy. *Journal of Ethics, Law, and Aging, 1,* 5–13.

Kayser-Jones, J., & Kapp, M. B. (1989). Advocacy for the mentally impaired elderly: A case study analysis. *American Journal of Law and Medicine, 14,* 353–376.

Lidz, C. W., Mulvey, E. P., Appelbaum, P. S., & Cleveland, S. (1989). Commitment: The consistency of clinicians and the use of legal standards. *American Journal of Psychiatry, 146,* 176–181.

Mahowald, M. B. (1993). When breaking may be keeping. In R. A. Kane and A. L. Caplan (Eds.), *Ethical conflicts in the management of home care: The case manager's dilemma,* pp. 168–175. New York, Springer Publishing Company.

Matthiesen, V., Lamb, K. V., McCann, J., Hollinger-Smith, L., & Walton, J. C. (1996). Hospital nurses' views about physical restraint use with older patients. *Journal of Gerontological Nursing, 22*(6), 8–16.

Miles, S. H., & Irvine, P. (1992). Deaths caused by physical restraints. *Gerontologist, 32*, 762–766.

Miles, S. H., & Meyers, R. (1994). Untying the elderly: 1989 to 1993 update. *Clinics in Geriatric Medicine, 10*, 513–525.

Monahan, J., & Steadman, H. J. (Eds.). (1994). *Violence and mental disorder: Developments in risk assessment.* Chicago: University of Chicago Press.

Morreim, E. H. (1994). Redefining quality by reassigning responsibility. *American Journal of Law and Medicine, 20*, 79–104.

Moss, R. J., and LaPuma, J. (1991, January/February). The ethics of mechanical restraints. *Hastings Center Report, 21*, 22–25.

National Council on Aging. (1988). *Care management standards—guidelines for practice.* Washington, DC: NCOA.

Olmstead v. United States, 277 U.S. 438 (1928).

Ossofsky, J. (1993). Untitled poem. *Gerontologist, 33*, 2.

Phillips, C. D., Hawes, C., & Fries, B. E. (1993). Reducing the use of physical restraints in nursing homes: Will it increase costs? *American Journal of Public Health, 83*, 342-348.

Post, S. G., & Whitehouse, P. J. (1995). Fairhill guidelines on ethics of the care of people with Alzheimer's disease: A clinical summary. *Journal of the American Geriatrics Society, 43*, 1423–1429.

Powderly, K. E. (1993). Process of legitimizing rule breaking. In R. A. Kane and A. L. Caplan (Eds.), *Ethical conflicts in the management of home care: The case manager's dilemma,* pp. 176–179. New York, Springer Publishing Company.

Raymond L., & Wentworth, B. (1993). Autonomy and safety: The client's perspective. *Topics in Geriatric Rehabilitation, 9*, 47–56.

Reigle, J. (guest ed.). (1996). Symposium on the use of restraints. *American Association of Critical Care Nurses (AACN) Clinical Issues, 7*, 571–635.

Robinson, B. E., Sucholeiki, R., and Schocken, D. D. (1993). Sudden death and resisted mechanical restraint: A case report. *Journal of the American Geriatrics Society, 41*, 424–425.

Rodin, J. (1986). Aging and health: Effects of the sense of control. *Science, 233*, 1271–1276.

Rubenstein, H. S., Miller, F. H., Postel, S., & Evans, H. B. (1983). Standards of medical care based on consensus rather than evidence: The case of routine bedrail use for the elderly. *Law, Medicine & Health Care, 11*, 271–276.

Sabatino, C. P., & Litvak, S. (1995). *Liability issues affecting consumer-directed personal assistance services.* Oakland, CA: World Institute on Disability and American Bar Association Commission on Legal Problems of the Elderly.

Schmidt, W. C., Jr. (1995). *Guardianship: The court of last resort for the elderly and disabled.* Durham, NC: Carolina Academic Press.

Schopp, R. F. (1991). The psychotherapist's duty to protect the public: The appropriate standard and the foundation in legal theory and empirical premises. *Nebraska Law Review, 70*, 327–360.

Stiegel, L. (1992). *Alternatives to guardianship—substantive training materials and module for professionals working with the elderly and persons with disabilities.* Washington, DC: American Bar Association Commission on Legal Problems of the Elderly.

Strumpf, N. E., & Evans, L. K. (1991). The ethical problems of prolonged physical restraint. *Journal of Gerontological Nursing, 17,* 27–30.

U.S. General Accounting Office. (1994). *Long-term care: Status of quality assurance and measurement in home and community- based services.* GAO / PEMD-94-19. Washington, DC.

U.S. General Accounting Office. (1993). *Long-term-care case management: State experiences and implications for federal policy.* GAO/HRD-93-52. Washington, DC.

Wilson, K. B. (1996). *Assisted living: Reconceptualizing regulation to meet consumers' needs and preferences.* Washington, DC: American Association of Retired Persons Public Policy Institute.

6

"A Dispirited Lot": Malpractice and What Else?

In an unprecedented move that paved the way for the consideration of similar policies in other states, the Massachusetts legislature in the summer of 1996 enacted legislation to give consumers easy access to data on every Massachusetts physician's malpractice awards, disciplinary actions by hospitals or medical boards, lawsuit settlements, and convictions for felonies or serious misdemeanors. To the majority of physicians there, publicizing their mistakes is just one more insult on top of what they perceive as managed care red tape, increasingly onerous insurance company and insurance purchaser scrutiny, and constant second-guessing from all sides. In a reaction typical of the state's medical profession, an internist in private practice for thirty-five years who is also a clinical professor of medicine complained, "We're a dispirited lot" (Carton, 1996).

Many American physicians in the twilight of the twentieth century are professionally dissatisfied. Although physician comments about, or emanating from, this unhappiness frequently center on attorneys and the awful negative impact of the medical malpractice system on the quality of American medicine for both patients and practitioners, the psychological malaise that runs throughout much of the medical profession today springs from a considerably more complicated combination of sources. The health care system and the role of the physician in it, having undergone a massive but orderly evolution over most of our history (Cassedy, 1991; Starr, 1982), has been swept up in a virtual revolution over the past decade and a half. This sea change in health care financing and delivery has created a whole slew of perceived ills.

As one English commentator (showing that this situation is not restricted to the United States) observed:

> All these new ills which plague both doctors and patients find their focus in the legal system. The fact that doctors, already stressed, are in addition placed in fear of a lawsuit whether they have done anything wrong or not, exacerbates a situation that is already tense and makes it intolerable. (McQuade, 1991)

According to other English medical leaders, "Doctors in most countries currently feel beleaguered" (Morrison & Smith, 1994, p. 1100).

This beleaguered feeling is instilled in physicians from the moment they enter medical school, if not before. According to a third-year medical student in his Honorable Mention-winning entry in the 1996 Alpha Omega Alpha Student Essay Competition:

> One can observe these days an undertone of resentment and increasing dissatisfaction among physicians. For the most part, this dissatisfaction has not been characterized fully, probably because few physicians have the time or inclination necessary to explore and analyze their increasing uncertainty. (Sandquist, 1996, p. 14)

This chapter briefly outlines some of the most pertinent sources of the current medical malaise. I look at how these factors manifest themselves as perceived ills that frequently find their focus in physician complaints about the legal system.

"NOT LIKE THE GOOD OLD DAYS": THE HEALTH CARE REVOLUTION

You Say You Want a Revolution? Why?

For the better part of two decades starting in the early 1960s, the medical climate in the United States formed what most physicians now over the age of thirty-five longingly refer to as "the good old days" of medical practice. Legislative creation of the Medicare and Medicaid programs and generous public appropriations for the Veterans Administration (now the Department of Veterans Affairs) and military health care systems, coupled with the blossoming of private indemnity insurance plans reimbursing both physicians and hospitals on a retrospective, fee-for-service basis and the development and proliferation of amazing technological advances in medicine, made the possession of a license to practice medicine—especially in a specialty or subspecialty—the virtual equivalent of a currency printing press. At the same time, external accountability for individual decisions made and actions taken in the context of patient care—including accountability through the medical malpractice system—was modest by any standards and absolutely quaint compared to the present environment. Few questions were asked either before or after treatments were rendered and payment was sent. What physician (or other health care provider, for that matter) wouldn't be nostalgic for such a golden age?

Unfortunately, though, by the early 1980s reality began its unwanted intrusion. A variety of important players in the health care marketplace began to believe (correctly, I think) (Kapp, 1989) that the existing ways in which we provided and paid for health care strongly overemphasized two fundamental social goals (namely, high quality of health care and broad accessibility of health services) to the extreme detriment of a third, equally important goal (namely, affordability). Put bluntly, our almost unbounded generosity had begun to result, in undeniable ways, in placing or keeping easy access to high-quality health services outside of the financial reach of many persons. This problem, largely unforeseen but eminently foreseeable, was threatening our continuing ability to provide both quality and access in a medically and ethically satisfactory manner.

Consumers, both individually and collectively (mainly through union membership) began to realize that dollars are fungible and that, therefore, a dollar spent by an employer to purchase health care for the employee, retiree, or dependent was a dollar consequently unavailable for salary or other fringe benefits. Moreover, deductible and coinsurance payments even for well-insured patients rose in amount or appeared for the first time. Employers, who are the primary purchasers of private health insurance in the United States, shifted more of the cost burden to employees and retirees by introducing or increasing the employee's/retiree's share of the premium payment for health insurance coverage, a practice that hit people directly in the wallet. Furthermore, the public became more sophisticated about the impact of rising health care costs on increases in the prices of all goods and services that needed to be purchased.

Government began to be concerned with uncontrolled health care costs in at least three distinct respects. First, it became concerned about the general inflationary and disruptive effect of continually rising health care costs on the American economy as a whole, an effect with huge potential political ramifications. Second, government is a major third-party payer for health care, through the federal (Medicare) and federal/state (Medicaid) entitlement programs and the federal (e.g., military health care, veterans' health care, the Indian Health Service, the Civilian Health and Medical Program of the Uniformed Services or CHAMPUS) and state (e.g., various public health programs) categorical health care programs. Rising health care costs with no end to the escalation in sight induced a long overdue fright into government in its payer role. Finally, the constellation of federal, state, and local governments function as employers and former employers of massive numbers of individuals for whom (and for whose dependents) governments *qua* employers purchase health insurance coverage. As costs rose, so too did the price of that coverage.

Commercial and nominally (but not really) not-for-profit health insurers (namely, Blue Cross and Blue Shield plans) began to worry as well. Previously these companies, acting in the role of money conduit between purchaser (usually an employer) and provider, with a little profit or excess capital margin built into the price, could react to increases in the cost of health care simply by raising premium prices. By the early 1980s, though, they began to realize that such a practice could not go on indefinitely. It became apparent that, in many cases, insurers were literally pricing themselves out of the market, as growing numbers of large corporations started to self-insure for health purposes rather than purchase coverage commercially and growing numbers of small companies either pooled resources to collectively self-insure or cut back on or dropped coverage for their employees, retirees, and dependents altogether. Health insurers found that to remain economically competitive in an increasingly sophisticated, demanding, and cost-conscious marketplace, they had a large stake in making health care more affordable (Miller, 1996).

As noted earlier, reflecting a phenomenon beginning shortly after World War II and continuing with questionable logic but substantial political support until today, most private health insurance in the United States is made available to workers, retirees, and dependents as a fringe benefit of employment. The national Internal Revenue Code encourages this arrangement by giving valuable tax advantages to both employers and employees who participate. Because of their enormous purchaser status, members of the business community became central players in many of the cost-containment initiatives of the past decade and a half. Corporations now understand that unrestrained health costs impair their relationships with their respective work forces by making it more difficult for them to give raises and to increase or even maintain other employment benefits. Unrestrained health costs also impair corporations' ability to remain economically competitive—especially in a global marketplace—when the prices they must charge for goods and services have to reflect the corporation's health insurance expenditures.

Finally, individual and corporate health care providers, including physicians, have belatedly and reluctantly gotten on the cost-containment bandwagon, ordinarily via the language of efficiency and effectiveness (Eddy, 1993). Providers' concerns in this sphere no doubt are driven in large part by a sincere desire to improve the quality of medical care and its accessibility and affordability by reducing waste and inefficiency. However, self-preservation cannot be discounted as another powerful factor here; most providers now understand that because consumers, governments, insurers, and employers all need (not just want, but need) to control health care costs, they (providers) must be actively involved in shaping the delivery and financing revolution lest its terms be dictated entirely without benefit of their meaningful insights.

What Hath the Revolution Wrought?

In light of the foregoing, by the middle of the 1980s the U.S. health care financing and delivery system had begun to change markedly, rapidly, and in many respects unpredictably. The Marcus Welby model of the individual, self-employed, fee-for-service practitioner dealing one-to-one with patients is now a dinosaur (Kletke, Emmons, & Gillis, 1996). The revolution continues at fuller tilt than ever today, with the private sector especially energized by the failure of President Clinton's comprehensive attempt in 1994 to redesign the American health care system through legislation and executive order (Aaron, 1996; Johnson & Broder, 1996).

Even a good rudimentary exposition of relevant changes would be well beyond the scope of this book, and a number of detailed explications of present and probable future strategic experiments and their underlying policy rationales are available elsewhere (e.g., Castro, 1994; Fuchs, 1993; Williams, 1995). Just a few of the most salient concepts that help to define the contours of the health care system at the outset of the new millennium are enumerated in cursory fashion next.

Prospective Payment

Although (driven primarily by cost concerns) an increasing amount of medical care today is delivered on an outpatient basis, hospitals have long been the centerpiece of most physicians' professional lives. As a leading medical historian put it bluntly but correctly, "Medicare gave hospitals a license to spend. The more expenditures they incurred, the more income they received—until the system was changed in the 1980s" (Stevens, 1989, p. 284). Under the previous system, hospitals were reimbursed by Medicare retrospectively (after-the-fact) for the costs they incurred in treating specific patients. Most private insurers and most states' Medicaid programs followed the federal government's lead. The perverse economic incentives at work in this arrangement are obvious, and hospitals responded accordingly: Admit as many patients as possible, extend their inpatient stays as long as possible, and treat as intensively (i.e., as expensively) as the patient could bear.

This money-making machine came to a halt (or so the health care industry exclaimed with panic at the time) with congressional enactment in 1983 of the Tax Equity and Fiscal Responsibility Act (TEFRA), which mandated future Medicare payments for inpatient hospital care under a newly designed Diagnosis Related Groups (DRG) scheme. In this new world order, which many private insurers and state Medicaid programs quickly adopted as their own payment schemes, payment rates for inpatient treatment were set ahead of time (prospectively) and were based not on the actual cost of care, but on the clinical reason for the particular patient's hospital admission. The theory was that, on the average, a patient's admitting diagnosis should predict the reasonable cost of care. If a hospital could treat the patient more cheaply than the prospective payment for the pertinent diagnosis, the hospital kept the difference; if treatment turned out to be more expensive, the hospital made up the deficit.

The financial incentives thus changed radically; hospitals now profit most by moving as much patient care as possible to their expanding outpatient components (where DRGs do not apply), discharging inpatients as quickly as feasible, and treating inpatients as efficiently and cost-effectively as possible. Although payments to physicians for their services, whether provided within or outside of the hospital, continue to be computed without reference to DRGs, the implications of the DRG system for practicing physicians are enormous. Previously the most valuable physicians for a hospital to have on its medical staff were the "heavy hitters" or "rainmakers" who admitted lots of patients, cultivated long lengths of stay, and treated patients as intensively as modern technology would permit. Under the post-1983 regime, the physicians just described became almost overnight precisely those with whom hospitals could least "afford" to be affiliated, and cost-conscious practitioners became the prize catches for one's medical staff. Hospitals have learned how to drive home that point to their physicians, who need hospital admitting and treatment privileges, in a variety of subtle and unsubtle ways intended to influence medical practice.

Managed Care

For physicians and other health care providers, the traditional retrospective, fee-for-service system of health services payment was profitable and autonomy-enhancing precisely because it was, in essence, *un*managed care. Although the United States had substantial experience with the opposite situation—that is, with various versions of managed care (Friedman, 1996)—it is only in the 1990s that managed care has taken the providers and consumers of the nation by storm.

Basically, managed care operates on the assumption that traditional fee-for-service, piecework financing provides disincentives for cost control and utilization management on the part of providers and patients. Managed care aims to reorganize financial incentives to discourage excessive and inappropriate utilization (Gold, Hurley, Lake, Ensor, & Berenson, 1995). Managed care is a generic classification for a wide range of organizational and financial arrangements that have evolved from the original concept of prepayment. The two main categories of managed care organizations (MCOs) at present, with infinite variations in detail under each heading, are health maintenance organizations (HMOs) and preferred provider organizations or arrangements (PPOs or PPAs).

As of July 1, 1995, fifty-four million Americans (21 percent of the population) were enrolled in 593 HMOs. There is a huge push currently by federal and state governments and private insurance companies to enroll Medicare and Medicaid beneficiaries into HMOs. Nearly three-fourths of all HMO enrollees were members of independent practice association (IPA) models, in which physicians, hospitals, and other entities contract with a health plan, or mixed models that involve more than one structure. Enrollment in more long-standing staff model HMOs, in which physicians are directly employed by the plan, was approximately 2 percent and declining. Of 340 HMOs reporting, 70 percent paid at least some primary care physicians through capitation (a specific, preset amount per patient, regardless of the patient's service utilization); half did the same for specialist physicians (Friedman, 1996, p. 957; Robinson & Casalino, 1995).

Preferred provider organizations or arrangements (PPOs/PPAs) are entities in which a limited number of health providers—physicians, hospitals, and others—agree to provide services to a defined group of people at a negotiated fee-for-service rate, which is usually less than their normal rate. There are incentives for enrolled people to use the preferred providers because the cost of services is fixed and bills are typically paid in full by the third-party payer. If the enrolled person goes to a nonpreferred provider, a lesser payment is made and the patient is responsible for the balance. Health care providers are willing (if not happy) to participate in these less-than-full-price arrangements in order to compete more effectively for a guaranteed share of the patient market. Purchasers of health insurance, mainly large employers, obviously are motivated by the ability to purchase coverage at less-than-full-price rates (Raffel & Raffel, 1994, pp. 66–67).

Clearly, one of the foremost objectives of managed care is to financially incentivize physicians to care for patients as inexpensively as possible, in part by reducing the length and intensity of services as compared with those that would have been provided under traditional fee-for-service cost maximization incentives. It is the managed care incentives exactly that many physicians (Berwick, 1996), as well as a number of legal and ethical observers (Malinowski, 1996), feel compromise good clinical diagnostic and therapeutic approaches and that therefore often place the physician in ethically and—it is believed—legally uncomfortable positions (Dalen, 1996; Sorum, 1996).

A theme commonly expressed by contemporary physicians is their feeling that they are skating on thin ethical ice every day with every patient because managed care forces them to compromise on the principle of best quality and safest care (Pierce, 1996, p. 974). For those physicians who believe that good clinical and ethical medicine is also the most effective risk management, there is the fear that managed care jeopardizes that equation. In accord with this view is Dr. Norman Levinsky (1996), who wrote that "managed care organizations introduce into the doctor-patient relationship powerful third parties whose economic goal is to limit medical care in order to reduce costs." Physicians express fear that the mutual trust and loyalty essential to an effective physician-patient relationship will be irreparably forfeited in this emerging climate (Emanuel & Dubler, 1995; Mechanic & Schlesinger, 1996; Orentlicher, 1995).

Many physicians lament, too, the negative impact of managed care on collegial relationships and the honoring of traditional ethical obligations among fellow physicians. Under managed care, its opponents claim, the specialist is given a strong incentive to induce the primary care physician to order as many tests and procedures as possible, so that the overuse profile compiled by the payer will reflect poorly on the primary care physician who did the ordering rather than on the specialist who used the test results and/or performed and got paid for the procedures.

At least one legal gadfly has responded to physician complaints with pronounced skepticism. George Annas (1996) claims:

> The reason physicians cannot fight against the market, now that the market is running medicine, is because there is no strong medical ethics core to the medical profession. Now doctors are often told what their profile is going to be. Doctors are now told how many patients they can see, what tests they can do, and what they can and cannot say to their patients. This is because doctors cannot credibly say, "I have professional ethics. There are some things I cannot do. I am a patient advocate. I have an ethical obligation to advocate for my patients. I must be loyal to my patients." Physicians should be able to say that, but they can't because they have not done it. This is at least partly because physicians have been given a blank check by the judiciary and by American society for the last twenty-five years, and they have used it to act irresponsibly. (p. 107)

Enhanced Quality Control, with Better Consumer Information and Involvement

Stemming both from financial pressures for more efficient and cost-effective medical care and from a more sincere concern about patient welfare, a variety of public and private strategies for assuring physician and institutional competencies have been developed or strengthened in recent years (Brennan & Berwick, 1996). These quality assurance strategies restrict in varying degrees the physician autonomy that in earlier times was virtually unbridled.

On the institutional level, among other things, state licensure, Medicare/Medicaid certification, and private accreditation standards and inspections have become more aggressive than before. In hospitals, for example, the Joint Commission on Accreditation of Healthcare Organizations (JCAHO) now looks closely at the institution's policies and procedures regarding restraint usage (see Chapter 5) and its process for resolving bioethical disputes. Faced with their imperative to demonstrate accountability, hospitals and other health care facilities, in turn, increasingly impose restrictions and requirements on physicians who have staff privileges or employment contracts. Cooperative team relationships among different providers who should be coordinating and rationalizing patient care are, quite predictably, a major casualty of this tense climate.

For individual physicians, besides pressures now brought in the name of quality assurance and improvement by corporate health care providers with whom they are affiliated, other modes of accountability multiply. These include, among numerous other things: more demanding and frequent licensure, relicensure, specialty board certification and recertification exams; more aggressive state medical boards under pressure from citizen advocacy watchdogs; the National Practitioner Data Bank created by the Health Care Quality Improvement Act of 1986, 42 United States Code §1101 *et seq.*; anti-fraud and abuse laws (Blumstein, 1996; Bucy, 1996); antitrust prohibitions; clinical laboratory regulations; and professional standards spelling out when a physician may accept a free lunch or calendar from a pharmaceutical company (Kapp, 1992). They all add up to a pervasive physician feeling that autonomy and control have been forfeited, and not even necessarily for any appreciable gain in quality anyway (Chassin, 1996).

Many of these initiatives have been based on the notion that making more information available to consumers is one of the best avenues to improved quality and accountability. As noted at the outset of this chapter, for instance, the Massachusetts legislature in 1996 enacted a law to give consumers ready access to a wealth of information about specific physicians practicing in that state. Groups like Consumers Union and the Public Citizen Health Research Group make data available in public libraries. Whereas some physicians welcome or are at least resigned to such developments, many others resent them as serious intrusions on physician privacy and freedom with little real corresponding benefit for the consumer. As one person in this camp protests:

> The practice of medicine is already being scrutinized very strictly in this country by a number of accredited bodies that establish the qualifications of each physician to practice medicine safely and efficiently. I do not believe a patient has any right to know my personal history, any more than I have the right to know the personal history of every airline pilot who flies me around or every cook or waiter who feeds me in a restaurant. Physicians and health care providers have rights, too. (Balducci, 1996)

STRANGERS IN THE OPPOSITE OF PARADISE: PHYSICIAN ATTITUDES IN THE CHANGING HEALTH CARE WORLD

For the large majority of physicians and their attitudes toward medical practice, implications of the foregoing developments in the health industry climate are decidedly not upbeat. Most physicians express a general sense of malaise among themselves and their peers about the changing organizational and financial climate of modern American medicine, consistent with the state of mind reflected in much of contemporary commentary in the professional literature (Hershey, McAloon, & Bertram, 1989; Hubbard, 1989, p. 330; Sprung & Eidelman, 1996, p. 731).

Many of today's physicians feel not only besieged by perverse economic incentives from within the health care system but also constantly hectored by external commentators who smear the ability and integrity of the medical profession in both the scholarly and popular media. The latter especially is perceived to push a thoughtless, reflexive "someone's head must roll" agenda for reporting the news about apparent medical mishaps. Critics promote a general accusation that patients need to be protected from their physicians in the modern era (Bobinski, 1994), given the inherent greed and conflicts of interest within the health care industry and among its players (Gray, 1991; Rodwin, 1993). Besides being told what to do by business managers and attorneys (Parmet, 1992), physicians find themselves sternly, publicly lectured about their confusing and unsettled ethical responsibilities to individual patients and to the larger society as the world changes around them (Wolf, 1994; Morreim, 1995). Physicians complain of being held simultaneously to multiple, inconsistent if not outright conflicting, more or less desirable and realistic standards of care—idealized, academic, practical, medicolegal, economic, managed care, and personal

(Argy, 1996), not to mention patient, expectations that may differ from all of these (Kellerman, 1996). At the same time, they are warned that "any ethic changeable by fortuitous social, economic, political, or legal fiat ultimately ceases to be a viable ethic" (Pellegrino, 1996, p. 1808).

THE UPSHOT: ROUND UP THE USUAL LAWYERS

The overall environment, then, is one within which physicians perceive themselves to be perpetually barraged with an unfair frontal attack on their personal incomes and their professional prerogatives. Within such an environment, what should we make of the sorts of physician complaints about lawyers and the medical malpractice specter that were described earlier in Chapters 1 and 2?

First, we must be aware that many physicians fear that conservative (i.e., less aggressive) patient care provided in response to managed care incentives to do less will often constitute poor-quality care that increases the physician's exposure to potential malpractice litigation and liability. For instance, physicians continually raise the ghost—bordering on mantra—of the well-publicized, more than a decade-old *Wickline v. State of California*, 288 Cal. Rptr. 661 (Cal. Ct. App. 1986), case as a paradigm of what literally petrifies them about being whipsawed today between malpractice attorneys and courts who have traditionally rewarded doing more, on one hand, and managed care accountants and utilization reviewers who reward doing less, on the other. The impact of *Wickline*'s influence on physician perceptions is instructive, because the overwhelming majority of physicians labor under a serious misunderstanding of the facts of this case.

Wickline involved a civil lawsuit brought against the California Medicaid agency by a patient who suffered an avoidable leg amputation, on the grounds that the agency's negligent prospective refusal to pay for the additional hospital days requested by the physician for observation purposes led directly to the patient's premature discharge and an exacerbation of the circulatory problems that necessitated the emergency amputation. Virtually every physician familiar with this case believes—quite inaccurately—that the attending physician was the main defendant in the lawsuit and was found liable for substantial monetary damages. In fact, the physician was not named in the complaint, because Mrs. Wickline viewed him as a friend and advocate. The Medicaid agency was exonerated on the grounds that the decision to discharge a patient may be made only by the physician, at least until all available appeals processes have been exhausted. Thus, the patient in *Wickline* recovered nothing from anyone. Nonetheless, this one case—with and indeed because of physicians' misinterpretations of it and because so far there is precious little other reported legal precedent with even tangential relevance—remains the doctors' lounge poster child for complaints about our legal system in the age of managed care (Pedroza, 1996).

The other oft-cited case in this area is *Wilson v. Blue Cross of Southern California* (1990). There, an appellate decision overturned a lower court's summary judgment that was based on *Wickline* dicta.

A comment commonly made by physicians is to the effect, "We would like to do our part to contain health care costs, but we feel shackled by the law." This sentiment is widely although not universally shared, as some physicians express hope that treatment guidelines developed by MCOs will have the positive effect of giving physicians the courage to resist unreasonable patient or family demands (see discussion of practice parameters in Chapter 7). Others share the opinion that forcing physicians to walk a tightrope balancing a variety of competing concerns may sharpen and invigorate analytical skills, compel better communication, encourage fuller exploration and development of alternatives, and otherwise dispel some of the intellectual sloppiness that often sneaks into the health care decision-making process in the absence of such tension. At the least, clear treatment guidelines emerging from managed care can reflect community values about what kinds of health care are worth providing to consumers (Loewy, 1996; U.S. General Accounting Office, 1996).

These minority-held hopes notwithstanding, a different kind of scenario is more usually cited by physicians as especially worrisome. This scenario involves the payer's denial of a submitted claim for payment for a test or procedure ordered by the physician, on the grounds that the particular intervention is deemed medically unnecessary by the insurer's utilization reviewer. Communication of a denial on this basis, physicians fear, has to make many patients question the physician's judgment and the propriety of the care being received. With the seeds of doubt thus planted in the patient's mind by the insurer or MCO, physicians fear widened exposure to litigation in the contingency of a bad patient outcome.

Another area of lamentation revolves around the amount of time that physicians are permitted by MCOs to spend with patients (and / or their families or other surrogates). Physicians widely express a sensation of being trapped by patient demands for their time but unable to fulfill those demands adequately and still comply with payment policies of insurers and MCOs. Knowing that patients and families who are disgruntled about the quality of the physician-patient relationship are the persons most likely to consult attorneys and bring lawsuits makes physicians particularly nervous about this situation.

At the same time, physicians' criticisms of the legal system's adverse repercussions for patient care may well represent the airing of more general frustrations with the larger perceived social and economic onslaught on medical practitioners. One prominent internist has written, "The insurance companies and Medicare have seen to it that our blood pressures rise every day when the mail is delivered, so fears of being sued have had to stand in line and wait their turn to get our attention" (Berczeller, 1994, p. 199). For many physicians, malpractice concerns take a back seat to managed care demons today because "at least law has a rationale." Additionally, even the most skittish physicians see only a portion of their patients as likely malpractice plaintiffs, whereas managed care forces the physician to talk with absolutely every patient about the financial ramifications of his or her medical recommendations.

A recent article in the AMA's newsletter is revealing. Enumerating the reasons that practicing medicine is no longer "fun," one physician member of the AMA Council on Ethical and Judicial Affairs listed worries about potential lawsuits threatening to "wipe out [his] financial security" first, but quickly followed that with lamentations about "having almost every medical decision questioned by some faceless employee at a computer terminal," "having a medication changed by the third-party payer because it is not on their formulary," "seeing longtime patients transfer to another physician because their employer could get a cheaper rate on health care coverage elsewhere," "large insurance companies and hospital corporations forming giant health care conglomerates, while antitrust regulations impede physicians from coming together as competitive entities in the new marketplace," and "all these changes, which increasingly constrain physicians' independence and question their judgment, also are taking away their sense of personal fulfillment" (Tenery, 1996).

Thus, physicians' unhappiness about their legal surroundings are just one piece (albeit an important one) of the entire picture. To what extent are legal anxieties only a lightning rod for physician unhappiness about that entire picture rather than an accurate focusing of physicians' true concerns? In a slightly different vein, to what extent are fears of medical malpractice being used to justify physician actions, such as early retirement from certain specialties, that would occur anyway but for different reasons?

THE PROOF OF THE PUDDING: WHAT WILL *REALLY* DRIVE MEDICAL CARE TOMORROW?

A substantial number of physicians speculate that despite their overall sense of dissatisfaction with the changing health care scene, at least one salutary effect may emerge from the present tumult. That would be a much clearer, more honest delineation of the actual impact of medical malpractice anxieties, versus the effects of other (mainly financial) forces, on the choices and behaviors of physicians in caring for patients. This is the pretext factor alluded to in the immediately preceding discussion.

At present, as noted in Chapter 2, it is unclear whether physicians' self-described defensive medicine practices have until now been induced by a true fear of potential litigation and liability or by the "do more" incentives of the fee-for-service payment system (Daly, 1995, pp. 102, 105). The former Congressional Office of Technology Assessment (OTA) suggested the latter, noting that fee-for-service policies and perceived legal risk management needs both push in the same direction of encouraging aggressive treatment (U.S. Congress, 1994, pp. 1, 15; U.S. Congress, 1993, pp. 18–19).

We may know considerably more about this issue—namely, whether medical behavior is motivated more by payment systems or by real legal anxieties—in the near future, as the financial and malpractice factors that purportedly influence physician behavior appear increasingly to be in tension with each other. A number of physicians and knowledgeable observers predict (Krieger, 1996; U.S. Congress, 1994, p. 94) that managed care's financial incentives for avoiding waste, inefficiency, and poor cost-effective choices are extremely likely to eliminate much of what is now labeled as defensive medicine. Ultimately, according to this view, direct, tangible, and immediate financial self-interest pointing toward restricting the amount and type of medical treatment made available to particular patients will trump the more indirect, remote, and indefinite possibility of adverse legal consequences for skimping on proper care (Woolhandler & Himmelstein, 1995).

Many physicians report that fear of Medicare/Medicaid chart audits (i.e., the daily presence of financial risk to the physician) is a significantly more powerful motivator of rethinking their care in specific cases than is the fear of liability exposure, which they understand is, even at its worst, a relatively rare event. Others indicate that most physicians currently are so focused on "whether they fit in as team players or they will have to start their own teams" that the remaining energy to worry about malpractice is seriously depleted. There also are accusations that contemporary attorneys are guilty of disrupting ethical medical practice not so much directly but more by complicity for failure to challenge stridently enough payers and reviewers who make decisions on the basis of inflexible, strict algorithms applied by bureaucrats of varied qualifications who sit far removed from the realities of patient care.

The speculation that financial concerns will clearly trump liability exposure worries may (and I believe will) turn out to be prescient; managed care and related financially motivated changes in how health care gets delivered and paid for may indeed be one answer to the defensive medicine problem. I turn to other potential solutions to that challenging phenomenon in the final chapter.

REFERENCES

Aaron, H. J. (1996). Health care reform: The clash of goals, facts, and ideology. In V. R. Fuchs (Ed.), *Individual and Social Responsibility*, pp. 107–141. Chicago: University of Chicago Press.

Annas, G. J. (1996). Facilitating choice: Judging the physician's role in abortion and suicide. *Quinnipiac Health Law Journal, 1*, 93–112.

Argy, O. (1996). Standards of care. *Journal of the American Medical Association, 275,* 1296.

Balducci, L. (1996). Barriers to patients' rights [Letter]. *New England Journal of Medicine, 335,* 136.

Berczeller, P. H. (1994). *Doctors and patients: What we feel about you.* New York: Macmillan Publishing Company.

Berwick, D. M. (1996). Payment by capitation and the quality of care. *New England Journal of Medicine, 335,* 1227–1231.

Blumstein, J. F. (1996). The fraud and abuse statute in an evolving health care marketplace: Life in the health care speakeasy. *American Journal of Law and Medicine, 22,* 205–231.

Bobinski, M. A. (1994). Autonomy and privacy: Protecting patients from their physicians. *University of Pittsburgh Law Review, 55,* 291–388.

Brennan, T. A., & Berwick, D. M. (1996). *New rules: Regulation, markets, and the quality of American health care.* San Francisco: Jossey-Bass.

Bucy, P. H. (1996). Crimes by health care providers. *University of Illinois Law Review, 3,* 589–665.

Carton, B. (1996, July 30). Massachusetts may publish data on doctors. *Wall Street Journal,* p. B1.

Cassedy, J. H. (1991). *Medicine in America: A short history.* Baltimore: Johns Hopkins University Press.

Castro, J. (1994). *The American way of health: How medicine is changing and what it means to you.* Boston: Little, Brown & Company.

Chassin, M. R. (1996). Improving the quality of care. *New England Journal of Medicine, 335,* 1060–1063.

Dalen, J. E. (1996). Managed competition: Who will win? Who will lose? *Archives of Internal Medicine, 156,* 2033–2035.

Daly, M. (1995). Attacking defensive medicine through the utilization of practice parameters: Panacea or placebo for the health care reform movement? *Journal of Legal Medicine, 16,* 101–132.

Eddy, D. M. (1993). Three battles to watch in the 1990s. *Journal of the American Medical Association, 270,* 520–526.

Emanuel, E., & Dubler, N. N. (1995). Preserving the physician-patient relationship in the era of managed care. *Journal of the American Medical Association, 273*, 323–329.

Friedman, E. (1996). Capitation, integration, and managed care: Lessons from early experiments. *Journal of the American Medical Association, 275*, 957–962.

Fuchs, V. R. (1993). *The future of health policy*. Cambridge, MA: Harvard University Press.

Gold, M. R., Hurley, R., Lake, T., Ensor, T., & Berenson, R. (1995). A national survey of the arrangements managed-care plans make with physicians. *New England Journal of Medicine, 333*, 1678–1683.

Gray, B. H. (1991). *The profit motive and patient care: The changing accountability of doctors and hospitals*. Cambridge, MA: Harvard University Press.

Hershey, C. O., McAloon, M. H., & Bertram, D. A. (1989). The new medical practice environment: Internists' view of the future. *Archives of Internal Medicine, 149*, 1745–1749.

Hubbard, F. P. (1989). The physicians' point of view concerning medical malpractice: A sociological perspective on the symbolic importance of "tort reform." *Georgia Law Review, 23*, 295–358.

Johnson, H., & Broder, D. S. (1996). *The system: The American way of politics at the breaking point*. Boston: Little, Brown & Company.

Kapp, M. B. (1992). Ethical issues in the relationship between American physicians and drug companies. *International Journal of Risk and Safety in Medicine, 3*, 73–80.

Kapp, M. B. (1989). Health care tradeoffs based on age: Ethically confronting the "R" word. *The Pharos, 52*, 2–7.

Kellerman, R. (1996). Another standard of care—the patient [Letter]. *Journal of the American Medical Association, 276*, 450.

Kletke, P. R., Emmons, D. W., & Gillis, K. D. (1996). Current trends in physicians' practice arrangements: From owners to employees. *Journal of the American Medical Association, 276*, 555–560.

Krieger, L. M. (1996). Reforming house staff's practice of defensive medicine. *Journal of the American Medical Association, 275*, 662af.

Levinsky, N. G. (1996). Social, institutional, and economic barriers to the exercise of patients' rights. *New England Journal of Medicine, 334*, 532–534.

Loewy, E. H. (1996). Guidelines, managed care, and ethics. *Archives of Internal Medicine, 156*, 2038–2040.

Malinowski, M. J. (1996). Capitation, advances in medical technology, and the advent of a new era in medical ethics. *American Journal of Law and Medicine, 22*, 331–360.

McQuade, J. S. (1991). The medical malpractice crisis—reflections on the alleged causes and proposed cures: Discussion paper. *Journal of the Royal Society of Medicine, 84*, 408–411.

Mechanic, D., & Schlesinger, M. (1996). The impact of managed care on patients' trust in medical care and their physicians. *Journal of the American Medical Association, 275*, 1693–1697.

Miller, I. (1996). *American health care blues: Blue Cross, HMOs, and pragmatic reform since 1960*. New Brunswick, NJ: Transaction Publishers.

Morreim, E. H. (1995). *Balancing act: The new medical ethics of medicine's new economics.* Washington, DC: Georgetown University Press.

Morrison, I., & Smith, R. (1994). The future of medicine. *British Medical Journal, 309,* 1099–1100.

Orentlicher, D. (1995). Health care reform and the patient-physician relationship. *Health Matrix, 5,* 141–180.

Parmet, W. E. (1992). The impact of health insurance reform on the law governing the physician-patient relationship. *Journal of the American Medical Association, 268,* 3468–3472.

Pedroza, K. R. (1996). Cutting fat or cutting corners: Health care delivery and its respondent effect on liability. *Arizona Law Review, 38,* 399–432.

Pellegrino, E. D. (1996). Ethics. *Journal of the American Medical Association, 275,* 1807–1809.

Pierce, E. C., Jr. (1996). Forty years behind the mask: Safety revisited. *Anesthesiology, 84,* 965–975.

Raffel, M. W., & Raffel, N. K. (1994). *The U.S. health system* (4th ed.). Albany, NY: Delmar Publishers.

Robinson, J. C., & Casalino, L. P. (1995). The growth of medical groups paid through capitation in California. *New England Journal of Medicine, 333,* 1684–1687.

Rodwin, M. A. (1993). *Medicine, money & morals: Physicians' conflicts of interest.* New York: Oxford University Press.

Sandquist, M. A. (1996, Fall). Do not go gently. *Pharos, 59,* 14–17.

Sorum, P. C. (1996). Ethical decision making in managed care. *Archives of Internal Medicine, 156,* 2041–2045.

Sprung, C. L., & Eidelman, L. A. (1996). Judicial intervention in medical decision-making: A failure of the medical system? *Critical Care Medicine, 24,* 730–732.

Starr, P. (1982). *The social transformation of American medicine.* New York: Basic Books.

Stevens, R. (1989). *In sickness and in wealth: American hospitals in the twentieth century.* New York: Basic Books.

Tenery, R. M., Jr. (1996, August 5). Who said medicine was supposed to be "fun"? *American Medical News,* p. 19.

U.S. Congress, Office of Technology Assessment. (1994). *Defensive medicine and medical malpractice.* Washington, DC: U.S. Government Printing Office.

U.S. Congress, Office of Technology Assessment. (1993). *Impact of legal reforms on medical malpractice costs.* Washington, DC: U.S. Government Printing Office.

U.S. General Accounting Office. (1996). *Practice guidelines: Managed care plans customize guidelines to meet local interests.* GAO/HEHS-96-95. Washington, DC.

Wickline v. State of California, 288 Cal. Rptr. 661 (Cal.Ct.App. 1986).

Williams, S. J. (1995). *Essentials of health services.* Albany, NY: Delmar Publishers.

Wilson v. Blue Cross of Southern California. (1990). 222 Cal.App.3d 660, 271 Cal. Rptr. 876.

Wolf, S. M. (1994, March–April). Health care reform and the future of physician ethics. *Hastings Center Report, 24,* 28–41.

Woolhandler, S., & Himmelstein, D. U. (1995). Extreme risk—the new corporate proposition for physicians. *New England Journal of Medicine, 333,* 1706–1708.

7

Reconciling Risk Management and Medical Ethics: Opportunities and Obstacles

A cartoon in the September 4, 1995, issue of the *New Yorker* depicts a physician sitting at his desk, speaking to a patient. In a remarkable display of candor (Kapp, 1993a), the physician is explaining, "I'll want to run a few tests on you, just to cover my ass." Whereas the general readership of that publication probably was amused, my strong guess is that most physicians I know would find that cartoon more sad or maddening than funny.

As the previous chapters illustrate in some depth, defensive medical practice is a subject with substantial ethical, legal, and social policy connotations. In law and policy, as well as medicine, the premier principle ought to be the same: "First, do no harm." Defensive medicine is no laughing matter precisely because, according to many, its various manifestations often result in harm to patients, their families, and others who deserve better. In this final chapter, I modestly explore some potential strategies for repairing the dynamic that too frequently leads from physicians' and other health care providers' fear of negative legal entanglements to the conduct of unethical medical practices that threaten to hurt exactly those vulnerable individuals whom both health care and legal professionals purport to help.

STRATEGIC APPROACHES TO DEFENSIVE MEDICINE

Tort and Other Legal Reforms

Most people who believe that the phenomenon of defensive medicine is both real and ethically harmful place most of the blame for this situation squarely on the shoulders of the legal system. Ironically but not too surprisingly, when asked for suggestions to address this situation, most of the critics respond in the same fashion that Americans typically have used to react to legal problems since our national beginnings (de Tocqueville, 1969); namely, they advocate enacting more "good" laws to overcome the negative consequences of those now in force. (The British, incidentally, are no better than Americans in this regard [Burn, 1996; Dyer, 1996], but I concentrate here on the United States).

The notion of holding medical practitioners accountable for their mistakes, despite the impression sometimes created by overhearing conversations in the physicians' lounge, is not the recent invention of a horde of hungry young attorneys on the prowl (although certainly today there are hordes of hungry young attorneys on the prowl). Rather, in the Babylonian legal code of Hammurabi in the second century B.C., medical providers were held strictly liable for death or injury of a patient and subjected to a specific menu of severe penalties. A surgeon who caused the death of a patient would have his fingers cut off; a nurse who mistakenly exchanged two infants had to sacrifice her breasts.

Without regard for this historical perspective, today almost every physician would quickly, indeed almost instinctively, react by naming tort reform if asked, "So, what should we do about defensive medicine?"–type questions. "Tort reform" in the 1990s is a large, ambiguous, and complex subject, and it is well beyond this book's scope to parse out in detail the various kinds of proposals for changing the civil justice system that have been enunciated by various groups and individuals, with differing degrees of legislative and judicial success (Kapp, 1990), in recent years; many good references are available for more background information (e.g., Weiler, 1995; Weiler, 1991; U.S. Department of Health and Human Services, 1987; Danzon, 1985). In this chapter, I deal at a more general level with the symbolic and pragmatic meanings of tort reform as a concept for members of the medical profession and their practices.

Many critics of the present defensive medicine scene (American College of Physicians, 1995) advocate—mainly at the national level—legislative initiatives that would both tinker with objectionable aspects of the traditional tort system for adjudicating medical malpractice claims and experiment with broader systemic kinds of changes. Advocates of these changes frequently phrase their support of these legislative experiments in terms of "basic fairness" to physicians now caught hard between the legal system and its threat of liability, on one side, and economic incentives driving physicians to limit care inappropriately, on the other (see Chapter 6). Proponents of this position call for systemic changes to counter the average physician's present malaise that the changing health care environment not only endangers the physician's role as patient advocate but also makes physicians feel they are being held responsible for decisions and outcomes that they no longer control. As one physician (who had recently been served with his first malpractice complaint after twenty years of spotless practice) told me, the main problem with the present tort system is the propensity of judges and juries to micromanage individual physician-patient relationships, with little if any thought to the impact of their decisions on the larger health care system or future relationships. He is correct in calling for "macro policies for macro problems."

In the tinkering category, the specific legislative alteration mentioned most frequently as likely to have a salutary impact on physicians' attitudes is placing caps or limits on the size of "outrageous" malpractice awards, especially for essentially speculative noneconomic (e.g., pain and suffering) and punitive damages. Other conventional tort reform measures that physicians list as important to them are: making a losing plaintiff pay the expenses of a prevailing defendant (a rule in place in virtually every other Western nation); setting limits on the amount of contingency fees allowable for plaintiffs' attorneys; and shortening statutes of limitation and tightening up their enforcement (e.g., eliminating the "discovery rule" that courts have created to effectively extend the time period for filing malpractice claims almost indefinitely).

Systemic changes proposed most often include no-fault mechanisms, in which payments for iatrogenic and nosocomial injuries would be paid out irrespective of the defendant's deviation from or compliance with acceptable professional standards (i.e., a Workers' Compensation model for patient injuries incurred in the course of receiving health care), and enterprise liability, under which employing agencies would be exclusively exposed to liability and individual physicians would be immune from malpractice lawsuits (Petersen, 1995). Mediation and other alternative dispute resolution (ADR) approaches that might reduce the apprehension of a protracted, public, and expensive adjudication process also are mentioned often as appealing to physicians.

Physicians and others who generally support different aspects of tort reform have a variety of reasons for taking this position. Most importantly, physicians claim that they desire the financial and psychological relief that they envision resulting from legislative changes that—among other benefits—reduce (a) the number of medical malpractice claims filed, (b) the percentage of malpractice claims concluding with payment to the plaintiff via settlement or jury verdict, (c) the size of payments when they occur, (d) the length and complexity of malpractice trials and appeals, and (e) (indirectly) the amount of professional liability insurance premiums.

The empirical evidence amassed thus far on the actual effects of tort reforms on the filing and disposition of medical malpractice claims is limited and fairly inconclusive (Bovbjerg, 1993; Kinney, 1995; Saks, 1992; Kapp, 1989a). Isolated studies appear periodically (Associated Press, 1996), but it is difficult to draw any definitive conclusions from them. As the *Wall Street Journal* has observed, in tort reform discussions, "much of the debate is driven by anecdote, and it doesn't seem to matter whether details can be verified" (Schmitt, 1995). Put bluntly, this is an arena in which our knowledge of what interventions really "work" is highly imperfect.

In any event, my chief purpose here is not to investigate whether tort reforms (or other types of interventions) are likely to accomplish the particular legal and economic objectives just enumerated. Nor am I asking directly whether these kinds of legal initiatives are likely to make physicians (and their families) happier with their lives and more satisfied with their careers. Rather, my main immediate question revolves around the degree to which various interventions might actually improve the ethical character of medical care provided to patients by inducing physicians to reduce the frequency of defensive practices that currently threaten or overwhelm good medical ethics. In other words, what is the probability that tort reform would change real physician behavior so as to improve the ethical content and character of the physician-patient relationship?

Predictions about such a causal connection between tort reform and positive behavioral change by physicians vary enormously among both practicing physicians and contributors to the professional literature. In its foray into this field, the Congressional Office of Technology Assessment (OTA) noted:

Predicting the impact of any malpractice reform on defensive medicine is very difficult, because there is little understanding of which specific aspects of the malpractice system actually drive physicians to practice defensively. Is it simply distaste for having one's actions judged by lay juries? Is it a desire to avoid court trials? Is it a fear, however unfounded, of being financially ruined? Or is it the belief that the legal standard of care is so capricious that the system offers no clear guidelines for how to avoid

liability? The relative importance of each of these factors in explaining motivations for defensive medicine will determine the effect of specific malpractice reforms on defensive medicine. (U.S. Congress, 1994, p. 10)

Moreover, an accurate prediction of changes in physician behavior would also need to take into careful account the pretext factor discussed at several earlier points in this book. Specifically, this means the extent to which anxiety about litigation and liability risks are publicly cited by physicians and other health care providers to try to justify their conduct that in truth is driven—whether consciously or not—by financial, psychological, cultural, and other nonlegal factors and incentives. A number of physicians hold a belief, and a larger number harbor at least the hope (although often with lukewarm confidence), that tort reform may make a meaningful impact on reducing the ethically undesirable aspects of defensive medicine practice. Some physicians surmise, for example, that tort reform would embolden emergency department physicians to reduce the excessive number of radiologic tests conducted on any patient—and especially children—who present with the slightest hint of head trauma.

A small group of commentators and researchers agree with this cautious optimism. In a sweeping exploration of new paradigms for health regulation in the United States, Brennan and Berwick (1996) suggest that with sufficient modification from the present scheme, "Tort litigation can be transformed into rational regulatory incentives" (p. 191). A recent Stanford University study compared hospital costs in states with different malpractice damage caps and concluded that "reducing clinicians' fears of malpractice can slash hospital expenditures by 5 percent for elderly patients with heart disease," presumably by reducing the amount of defensive medicine practiced, without making those patients any sicker (Kessler & McClellan, 1996). An earlier study suggested that with fear of liability eliminated from the equation, physicians are more willing to withdraw life-sustaining medical interventions from dying patients in accordance with the wishes of relevant participants and the broad social and professional consensus on ethical practice (Perkins, Bauer, Hazuda, & Schoolfield, 1990) (see Chapter 4). The results of my own study of the impact of Ohio's 1990 advance directive statute, however, supports an opposite interpretation, namely, that the practices of many physicians in end-of-life scenarios are rather independent of current law (Kapp, 1996).

A central problem may well be that the facts—that is, the actual impact of tort reforms on the number and outcome of filed malpractice claims—too often are close to irrelevant in determining physician behavior. For most physicians, tort reform is much more a symbolic than a pragmatic matter. In other words, in this emotionally charged atmosphere, tort reform's value derives more from its reaffirmation of the physician's privileged role in society—from its letting physicians feel positive about themselves, their work, and their patients—than from any specific tangible impact on the process or outcomes of litigation (Hubbard, 1989, pp. 296–297).

At the same time, a substantial number of physicians confide that although they personally support tort reform because of its anticipated financial and psychological benefits for physicians, they would discount the probability of tort reform producing any serious effect in terms of reducing the conduct of defensive medicine practices that carry negative ethical implications for patient care. Members of this group describe themselves and their medical colleagues as "creatures of habit," driven in reality by a panoply of other factors besides legal risk perceptions, in whose professional behavior tort reform might at best make a small dent. These participants caution that medical practice evolves slowly and that "old schools" of practice are excruciatingly difficult to change.

The pessimists (or realists, depending on one's view) opine that tort reform cannot improve physician behavior as long as there are financial incentives to practice defensively. Additionally, for many physicians, zero tolerance of legal risk is the gold standard, and hence *any* exposure to litigation, let alone liability, whatsoever is too great a force not to dominate their practice. As long as physicians believe that there are "swarms of attorneys buzzing around in search of patients with bad outcomes," anything short of total and unconditional advance immunity will be insufficient to alleviate physician anxiety enough to change practice patterns.

(This quest for absolute immunity from legal consequences as a condition of rendering good medical care, incidentally, is nothing new or provincial. It dates back at least to physicians practicing in ancient Greece [Lascaratos & Dalla-Vorgia, 1996]).

Some attorneys are even skeptical that physicians would really believe, and therefore be influenced in their conduct by, complete statutory immunity anyway. This skepticism is supported by evidence derived over the past couple of decades showing that enactment of Good Samaritan statutes in every American jurisdiction, making it almost impossible to successfully sue a physician (or anyone else, for that matter) for rendering aid in an emergency situation (e.g., roadside automobile accidents), has had absolutely no impact—positive or negative—on physicians' willingness to render such aid (Dillard, 1995). Similarly, statutes have been enacted in Virginia (Va Code ch. 1, Title 54.1-1.06, §32.1-127.3), Utah (§58-12-3.5), North Carolina (GS 90-21.14,

§1), Florida (§766.1115), Kentucky (Ky Rev Stat ch 42), South Carolina (§33-55-210), Iowa (§641-88.1-88.14), and elsewhere to provide legal immunity to physicians who serve uninsured indigent patients. The demonstrated impact of these statutes on the willingness of physicians to volunteer such care, however, has been nil. Obviously, other factors besides fear of legal liability are at play.

Some observers complain that organized medicine demands not just fair, but preferential legal treatment of physicians and that "it [organized medicine] will not rest as long as liability remains even a blip on the screen." The public policy issue, according to this view, is how much special treatment legislators are willing to afford to physicians and what political concessions will be extracted from the medical profession in return. Under this view, organized medicine likely will be thrown a few more "bones" in order to co-opt its support on larger issues (Annas, 1996, p. 107).

Many individuals suggest that tort reform legislation might make some difference in physician behavior only if physicians really believe, emotionally as well as intellectually, that their own legal risks are thereby greatly reduced. The clearest signal in this regard would be sent in the form of lowered liability insurance premiums for a sustained period of time. Premium price reductions unambiguously connected to tort reforms might be the most powerful way to get the message across to physicians that it is "okay to pull back" on defensive medicine and "to think again about quality." Overall, most physicians agree that the actual effects of tort reforms would depend most heavily on how those reforms were portrayed and packaged in the medical community; here as elsewhere, public relations carries more weight than does substance.

There exist several other ideas for productive legal reforms. A number of participants in the health care system have called for clearer, less ambiguous, more concise guidance within the letter of the law itself about acceptable physician conduct (Quill, 1994, p. 707). Stated sharply, "Laws should promote perfection in practice, not on paper."

One leading expert in the field of medical errors advocates a system, modeled on the one used by the Federal Aviation Administration for preventing and remedying safety problems in aircraft, in which a person who reports medical errors would be immune from any legal liability associated with the error reported (Leape, 1994, p. 1857). Another analyst states, "It is imperative that an atmosphere be created in which medical care personnel can freely provide data about errors and near errors they experience" (Bogner, 1994, p. 379). This proposal is built on the theory that, ironically, talking about mistakes ordinarily is excellent long-range risk management because the discussion may lead to important, needed improvements in practice (Christensen, Levinson,

& Dunn, 1992, p. 430). Forgiveness encourages "help-seeking" behavior (Bosk, 1979, p. 178). "We need to know why good doctors sometimes make bad mistakes. . . . We owe it to our patients and to ourselves to increase our knowledge about mistakes" (Ely, 1996). A path-breaking conference was held in October 1996 in Rancho Mirage, California, on the subject of "Errors in Health Care" (Prager, 1996). Convened by the American Medical Association, American Association for the Advancement of Science, Joint Commission on Accreditation of Healthcare Organizations, and the Annenberg Center for Health Sciences, with support from numerous other organizations, this three-day meeting brought together national experts from the fields of medicine, law, bioethics, management, and health services research. The goal was to give impetus to a process dedicated to fashioning, and then implementing, a major national agenda on prevention, education, and research regarding errors in patient care.

As noted in Chapter 1, the not infrequent occurrence of errors, sometimes serious in their implications for patient safety and welfare, in the delivery of health care is a problem that has long been recognized (Bosk, 1979; Hilfiker, 1984; Leape, 1994). A number of scattered initiatives to address this state of affairs have been launched over the years (American Society of Health-System Pharmacists, 1995; Howard, Gaba, Fish, Yang, & Sarnquist, 1992). In recent years, though, well-publicized statistical analyses (Physician Insurers Association of America, 1996; Bates, Leape, & Petrycki, 1993) and individual stories regarding lives jeopardized or diminished by health system errors have greatly increased both public and professional acknowledgment and concern about this matter.

As already alluded to, purported prophylactic/corrective strategies such as voluntary accreditation and medical malpractice tort law appear to have been largely ineffective in achieving their quality assurance goals and may even exacerbate the problem in some cases. For instance, the reluctance of key actors to admit, even to their colleagues, and remedy their mistakes in a timely and honest manner is—so they believe, at least—"reinforced by the American tort system" (Levy, 1995, p. 39) and translated into a harmful "Code of Silence." Consequently, substantial consensus that the time has arrived for a more decisive and coordinated plan of action inspired the Fall 1996 gathering on medical errors.

Among other things emanating from that conference, the AMA unveiled its National Patient Safety Foundation, which "embraces the idea that quality is the result of a continuous process, in which the number of errors can be reduced by understanding and examining the systems in which medical care is delivered. The foundation's goal is to promote a national patient safety movement in which awareness of potential mistakes is a part of every medical interaction and setting" (Seal of approval, 1996). Other organizations are similarly involved in this quest (Figure 7.1).

Other ideas often raised include proposals for (a) more emphasis on physician self-regulation as part of a continuous recertification process including a clinical component and (b) eliminating penalties just because a physician has been sued. For instance, states should remove questions about lawsuits from medical relicensure questionnaires.

A substantial number of commentators urge that tort reform and other legal interventions aimed at reducing the liability specter for physicians be considered seriously only if those changes are incorporated as part of a comprehensive, systemic overhaul of health care delivery and financing in the United States. In this way, quality oversight of physicians could move from the disorganized "spot checking" of the current malpractice system to scrutiny and enforcement at the level of the particular health plan. Those who endorse broad systemic revisions would insist on adequate mechanisms for quality assurance and for compensating injured patients (especially vulnerable patients such as those in nursing facilities and hospices whom the current system probably protects inadequately) as necessary preconditions to major tort changes.

Figure 7.1
Sample of Organizations Involved in Addressing Errors in Health Care.

Anesthesia Patient Safety Foundation
Room 9564 Ermire Building, Mercy Hospital
1400 Locust Street
Pittsburgh, PA 15219-5166

Institute for Safe Medical Practices
320 W. Street Road
Warminster, PA

Institute for Healthcare Improvement
135 Francis Street
Boston, MA

National Council on Patient Information and Education
Suite 810
666 Eleventh Street, NW
Washington, DC 20001-4542

On the whole, purported legal solutions to the defensive medicine problem must be examined with caution. As physician/attorney David Orentlicher (1994a) reminds us, even the best laws cannot get us around the fact that physician behavior ultimately is driven by the particular physician's values (pp. 1301–1302). Thus, tort reform is a potential double-edged sword. To the extent that physicians perceive legal reforms as sheltering them, they may make positive practice changes accordingly; but if, on the other hand, legal anxieties really are a pretext or camouflage for doing things the physician prefers to do anyway, physicians will continue present behavior patterns regardless of legal system changes. Although in some places he has advocated direct command and control regulation as the only effective method of changing physician behavior ("to the extent that law continues to dominate medical ethics in the United States, changes in the ethical behavior of physicians will continue to require legal action" [Annas, 1995, p. S14]) leading medicolegal commentator George Annas also has quoted with approval former *New England Journal of Medicine* editor Dr. Franz J. Ingelfinger's admonition that if physicians keep turning to the courts to resolve medical matters, physicians' dependence on lawyers and the law can only get worse (Annas, 1994, p. 1542). The same comment would apply to physicians turning to the legislatures for solutions, and it explains the essentially Catch-22 quality of tort reform efforts, at least to date.

Education about the Law

Many of the most active physicians in this arena, as well as almost all of the scholarly commentators, spend a good portion of their professional lives in academic settings. It is no wonder, then, that more and better education of physicians about law and the American legal system is frequently cited as a strategy for addressing the tension between defensive medicine and ethical practice. (Medical and legal leaders abroad also have called for education about the interface between medicine and law as a way to help members of both professions see matters better from the patient's perspective [Richards, Kennedy, & Woolf, 1996]).

In at least one study, legal defensiveness appeared to be lower among experienced clinicians than more novice physicians, a fact interpreted to indicate that the more a physician understands about both clinical matters and the law, the better in terms of behavior (McCrary, Swanson, Perkins, & Winslade, 1992). The authors of that study recommend that "physicians obtain their information regarding such law from appropriate sources such as academic lawyers in medical schools or health law institutes, bioethicists, and other sufficiently knowledgeable members of ethics advisory committees. Other physicians should only be regarded as appropriate sources of knowledge if they have graduate-level legal training or substantial expertise in the areas of law pertaining to bioethics" (p. 375).

Medical schools and residency programs report substantial educational efforts today in the realm of law and the legal system (Williams & Winslade, 1995). One must be curious about the lasting value of these efforts, though, when so many physicians complain emphatically about the *paucity* (or so they perceive) of opportunities for decent legal education by medical students and residents in current training and the need to do much more in this regard. In addition, a number of commentators have questioned the positive impact of education on the behavior of persons who do not evaluate their own legal risks rationally; "cognitive psychology reveals that we are likely to overestimate tort risks and avoid desirable activity" (Shuman, 1993, p. 166). To the extent that physician behavior is driven by what are sometimes described as "urban legends," continuing education will not accomplish anything as long as there exists even the most remote basis for believing any of those legends.

Others are skeptical about the willingness of practicing physicians and those in training to devote the necessary time and effort to reading legitimate literature or attending and paying attention to appropriate educational sessions in legal medicine in light of the many other pressing demands on their time and energy. Still others express doubt that education can overcome physicians' innate phobia about the law, which has been described as "like a fear of water for the nonswimmer." Put bluntly, "Facts are no match for free-floating fears."

Some skeptics of the likely success of continuing education efforts (especially in the form of balanced, objective articles in major medical journals) for the rank-and-file members of the medical profession support making such efforts nonetheless, but urge that they be directed to the medical "elites." Under this approach, enlightenment of leaders in medical education and organized medicine ("the generals"), who ought to be the most educable about medicolegal concepts, would exert a slow but sure ripple effect on the knowledge and attitudes of the medical infantry.

To the extent that it does have practicality and worth, continuing education should enlighten physicians and other health professionals about both substantive (e.g., applied statistics about the usefulness of screening tests) and procedural (e.g., who to include in discussions) facets of medical decision making. Legal risks, rights, and responsibilities must be put into realistic perspective, so that knowledge and judgment supplant the familiar mantra of "but I can be sued." Advisors (e.g., risk managers and attorneys—see Chapter 3) must be educated to function as enablers and supporters instead of paid paranoids. We should be able to expect a high degree of introspection and truthfulness from physicians and other health professionals and administrators about the real reasons for their practices, as opposed to automatically scapegoating the legal system for every questionable action, and it should also be a duty on their part to inquire and complain further when a perceived rule "is understood to work against good care" (Johnson, 1993, p. 77). Education about ethical principles should aim at providing a flexible yet substantial set of guidelines for analyzing and acting upon a set of facts and hence overcoming the "every case is different" syndrome that too frequently serves merely as a convenient pretext for issue avoidance.

Even done properly, legal education of physicians may take a generation to change behavior for the better. The current "folklore" will need to die out, and will do so slowly as long as there are senior physicians passing down horror stories and undoing any value of formal education to which the student, resident, or newer attending physician is simultaneously exposed. This dynamic can be fixed only when senior physicians, to whom the less experienced look up as mentors and role models, are teaching in tandem with, rather than in opposition to, properly knowledgeable teachers who know the legal system. This transformation in medical education will not take place overnight.

Risk Management Education

Closely related but not identical to education about applicable law and the legal system is instruction about effective risk management principles and strategies. A number of physicians and administrators put substantial weight on the value of educating physicians that risk management need not—and indeed should not—compromise principles of ethical clinical practice. Most medical malpractice lawsuits originate with the patient's or family's dissatisfaction with the physician's interpersonal behavior, especially perceived communication and access problems (Levinson, Roter, Mullooly, Dull, & Frankel, 1997; Hickson, Clayton, Entman, Miller, Githens, Whetten-Goldstein, & Sloan, 1994). Stupid, uncontroversial mistakes like the medical office's failure to notify patients about abnormal test results are both bad ethics and fodder for legal claims (Boohaker, Ward, Uman, & McCarthy, 1996). Rather than compel physicians toward "do everything" practice patterns whose legal benefit is largely illusory, constructively presented risk management education ought to stress better communication within the health care team and between team members and the patient/family (Levinson, 1994), positive provider–patient/family relationships generally, and accurate and complete documentation as the keys to effective litigation and liability risk reduction.

I fully concur with the physician who told me, "The logic of physicians who gear their practice patterns in ways they think are negative in order to protect themselves legally is false and circular. It is far less risky to explain one's decisions and actions better to the patient and the chart than to consciously practice bad medicine."

Many malpractice analysts talk about the potential proactive role of risk management education (Frisch, Charles, Gibbons, & Hedeker, 1995; Morrissey, 1996), often advocating mandatory continuing education in this area. The states of Florida and Massachusetts already impose such a requirement for physicians, although "risk management" is defined so broadly in their regulations that the educational impact may get somewhat diluted. Substantiation of formal risk management's salutary impact on liability experience is beginning to emerge from the best source of data in this sphere, namely, the insurance industry (MMI Companies, 1996).

Clinical Practice Parameters

Over the past decade, one aspect of the changing health care scene that has evoked a substantial amount of controversy in the area of liability risk and physician behavior is the expanding development of clinical practice parameters (Taler, 1996). Although there is some variation among members of different medical specialties, a sizable majority of physicians appear to endorse this development, at least in theory. It is a very important potential means of changing physician behavior in a way that should improve the clinical quality of care and the ethical character of the physician-patient relationship, while providing physicians with salutary benefits by reducing legal liability exposure. "Professional guidelines [provide a frame of reference for the physician in any particular clinical circumstance but still] offer greater flexibility than legal regulations in implementing standards and would also serve as a restraint on an impetus to testing [or other unnecessary intervention] from malpractice litigation" (Wertz, Fanos, & Reilly, 1994, p. 880). However, these positive impacts will occur only if (and as we shall see quite shortly, this is an enormous "if") individual practitioners actively "buy into" the validity and value of practice parameters.

The proliferation of clinical practice parameters is an international phenomenon (North of England Asthma Guideline Development Group, 1996). In the United States, a growing array of government agencies, particularly the federal Agency for Health Care Policy and Research (AHCPR) (Crowley, 1994, pp. 385–388), and professional organizations including the American Medical Association (AMA) through its Physician Performance Assessment Program (Seal of approval, 1996) and the American Medical Directors Association's Clinical Practice Guidelines Project on depression, heart failure, pressure ulcers, and urinary incontinence (Anonymous, 1996) are plunging into the business of creating and disseminating varied versions of clinical practice guidelines. So, too, are specialty societies (Katz & Ouslander, 1996), payers, ad hoc panels, and individual health care provider entities (Webster, 1995).

The 1996 annual AMA compilation lists approximately eighteen hundred different guidelines or parameters, including four hundred added since the previous year (American Medical Association, 1996). In addition to "clinical practice parameters," the phenomenon under discussion here also has been referred to variously as practice guidelines, practice standards, critical pathways (Butler, 1995), and an array of other labels. Though the terminology in this arena has frequently been confused and confusing, for our purposes clinical practice parameters (CPPs) will convey the concept adequately.

CPPs are written strategies for patient management, developed to assist physicians in clinical decision making. Ideally based on a thorough evaluation of the scientific literature and relevant clinical experience, CPPs describe the range of acceptable approaches to diagnose, manage, or prevent specific diseases or conditions. CPPs are educational tools that enable physicians to obtain the advice of recognized clinical experts, stay abreast of the latest clinical research, and assess the clinical significance of often conflicting research findings. When properly constructed and disseminated, CPPs provide a rational basis for continuous quality assurance and improvement, utilization review, facility accreditation, physician staff privileging, decisions by managed care organizations about particular physicians' continued participation, and other review activities (Field & Lohr, 1990).

Impetus for Development

The impetus behind the current burst of activity in CPP development is threefold. First, significant variations in clinical practice exist among different physicians, without any sufficient explanation for those variations based on patient conditions. CPPs have the potential to improve the quality of patient care by reducing medically unjustified outlier practice. Second, given the current national concern about attaining demonstrable value (positive outcomes) for money spent on health care, some argue that CPPs can be an effective mechanism for eliminating or reducing inappropriate, unproven practices and thus controlling costs without impairing quality of care. Third, dissatisfaction with the present American legal system for resolving claims of medical malpractice is widespread, and the prospective guidance (i.e., greater predictability in the applicable legal standard of care [U.S. Congress, 1994, pp. 17–18]) that CPPs offer physicians appears to be a preferable strategy for avoiding medical mishaps in the first place and adjudicating fault in cases where mishaps do occur.

To many, CPPs are an appealing alternative to the status quo, which entails continued use of largely nonvalidated medical practices, with consequent substantial variations among practitioners (Reid, Lachs, & Feinstein, 1995); uncontrolled (or at least unsustainably expensive) health care costs with little or no demonstrable relationship between amount spent and quality attained; and a system of malpractice litigation based on ad hoc, retrospective determinations of negligence, influenced by evidentiary swearing contests between hired experts (McConkey, 1995). Given the sharp contrast between the potential benefits of CPPs and the proven weaknesses of past and current approaches to issues of quality, cost control, and malpractice lawsuit prevention and adjudication, there is a growing consensus that continued tinkering with "the Theory of Bad Apples" (Berwick, 1989) is unacceptable. Instead, further development and dissemination of CPPs is inevitable and has received endorsement from influential quarters (Physician Payment Review Commission, 1994, pp. 296–297).

Predicting the actual long-range effects, if any, of the CPP movement on physicians' ability to avoid, or if necessary defend themselves in, malpractice claims (or against criminal prosecutions [Capron, 1995, p. 27]) is still a highly speculative exercise, with practitioners and commentators falling into both optimistic (Hall, 1991; Rosoff, 1995) and pessimistic camps. For the time being, the majority of current practicing physicians are likely to lean toward the latter position. However, CPPs no doubt have the greatest chance of influencing the practices of physicians who honestly wish to practice quality, ethical medicine but who now are reluctantly influenced in a negative way by a sincere anxiety about legal liability.

Existing data on the subject of legal ramifications are preliminary and inconclusive (Hyams, Brandenburg, Lipsitz, & Brennan, 1995). Nonetheless, I can at least usefully outline both the potential salutary effects as well as possible dangers and problems associated with the proliferation of CPPs and suggest briefly some strategies to increase the positive effects (Brown & Procopio, 1995; Kapp, 1995; Kapp, 1993b; National Health Lawyers Association, 1995; Rinella, 1995).

Possible Positive Impacts

First, a civil claim (of which medical malpractice is one type) based on a theory of negligence requires the plaintiff to prove that the defendant proximately or directly caused the plaintiff injury by deviating from acceptable standards of care (Boumil & Elias, 1995, p. 1). If CPPs succeed in improving the quality of patient care by reducing inappropriate, unproven physician practices, a natural result should be a reduction in bad patient outcomes directly due to medical interventions, with a consequent reduction in malpractice claims.

Second, CPPs have the potential to discourage plaintiffs' attorneys who work on a contingency fee arrangement from filing malpractice claims in situations where the patient has suffered some iatrogenic or nosocomial harm despite the provider's compliance with applicable CPPs. Those attorneys presumably would reject cases in which they believe that the provider's compliance with pertinent CPPs would make it extremely difficult to meet the plaintiff's burden of proving the provider's deviation from the acceptable practice standard.

Third, in a related vein, the fact of physician compliance with relevant CPPs ought to be powerful support in the defense of malpractice claims that do get filed. Depending on each jurisdiction's evolving judicial precedent and legislative or regulatory enactments, the defendant's compliance with relevant CPPs should be introducible at trial as either *some* valid evidence of conformity with the proper standard of practice (i.e., for its persuasive weight) or as *conclusive* proof of the correct standard. A legislatively created demonstration project in Maine has attempted to gather data (albeit with little success thus far) regarding the impact of making compliance with official CPPs available as a defense in malpractice cases on the filing rates and ultimate outcomes of malpractice claims, as well as the impact on clinical practice. Several other states also are experimenting in this arena, and Bill Clinton's unsuccessful 1994 Health Security Act proposal (Johnson & Broder, 1996) would have authorized federal sponsorship of pilot demonstration projects to encourage and evaluate the use of CPPs.

Potential Dangers and Problems

Despite the number of parameters and similar documents presently extant, in many respects this is an enterprise still very much in its early stages. Therefore, it is essential to identify and address a number of potential problems that, if not anticipated and attended to in a timely fashion, could seriously jeopardize the risk management value of CPPs or, worse yet, increase physician exposure to liability risk. First, some CPPs may be poorly drafted. For instance, they may be based more on political considerations within particular professional organizations than on scientific evidence, or they may be confusingly or ambiguously worded and either too detailed or too general. Specific CPPs may be suspect because they are developed and disseminated prematurely, that is, before sufficient scientific data are generated on which a professional consensus can intelligently be predicated. The generation of adequate evidence ought logically to precede the drafting of evidence-based CPPs (Komaroff, 1987; Sarwar, 1996). CPPs that are poorly drafted in any of these respects or for any of these reasons may end up doing more harm than good for both patients and their health care providers.

Second, when various entities promulgate CPPs in the same subject area, inconsistencies and even outright contradictions may occur. Practitioners are then confronted with the dilemma of how to reconcile these nonidentical or conflicting sources and with the need to choose among them in actual patient treatment. The recent national debate among leading professional organizations over age guidelines for routine periodic cholesterol screening for healthy people sharply illustrates this practical conundrum (Hearn, 1996).

Another potential problem with CPPs is the possible misinterpretation and misuse of them by the courts or other adjudicative bodies. The confusion created in the mid-1980s when Medicare and other third-party payers took a diagnosis-related-group (DRG) methodology developed for clinical purposes and constructed a new payment schema around it is a prime example of how extended application can cause problems. At the same time, the possibility of CPP misuse in no way ought to discourage practitioners' enthusiasm about CPPs when they are used properly. To prevent misuse or misinterpretation of CPPs, entities developing these documents should state the CPPs' purposes clearly and frequently and communicate this information to all potential users and beneficiaries.

Probably the most potentially devastating liability-related danger associated with CPPs concerns the problem of physician noncompliance with relevant CPPs without adequate justification of that deviation and accompanying documentation. Certainly, it is in practitioners' best interests to be aware of CPPs available to them and to be familiar with their content and use. The biggest threat to physicians facing lawsuits involving CPPs occurs when the plaintiff's attorneys know more about the guidelines than the physicians do.

Physician Noncompliance

Thus far, although there appears to be some variation by geography and medical specialty, CPPs generally have done little to change actual physician behavior (Ellrodt, Connor, Riedinger, & Weingarten, 1995; Kadzielski, Weingarten, & Schroder, 1995; Schriger, 1996). In light of the continuing theoretical popularity and tangible development of CPPs, the potential legal ramifications of these documents for physicians, and the possible benefits to patients through better clinical and thereby more ethical care from physicians, careful scrutiny of the origins of, and the obstacles to (Schwartz & Shulkin, 1995; U.S. Congress, 1994, pp. 18, 92), better physician compliance is imperative, as is the consideration of effective intervention strategies.

Many factors influence physician practice patterns (Allery, Owen, & Robling, 1997). Two forces, however, are likely to predominate in the etiology of medical conduct—namely, (a) most physicians are heavily influenced by the real or perceived practice patterns of their respected professional peers and try to emulate those patterns, and (b) physicians are especially driven by personal intuitive interpretations of their own recent experiences in treating patients (the "my last case" syndrome). For many physicians, in fact, the "last case"—especially when the resulting experience was negative—exerts a far more powerful and continuing impact on the physician's future behavior than do scientific evidence and reasoning; the logic of one's own experience determines the perceived usefulness of others' research. Put differently, scientific evidence takes its meaning only in the light of the current clinical situation and past clinical experience; foremost, physicians trust their personal experiences (Bosk, 1979, pp. 45, 85–87, 89, 92).

Against this challenging background, CPPs aim to influence or change physician behavior. First, CPPs attempt to convey information that will alter physician beliefs about which practices are likely to produce the most favorable patient outcomes. This is backed up by the threat of financial and legal sanctions for unjustified or insufficiently documented physician noncompliance. When all of the forces integral to health care delivery—clinical, financial, and legal—push in the same direction, they are most powerful in influencing physician behavior (Orentlicher, 1994b, pp. 598–605). Conversely, a health care delivery system (or more accurately, health care delivery marketplace) that sends mixed or even conflicting incentive messages to physicians is destined to fail. In sum, physicians are most likely to act consistent with what they perceive to be their own best interests.

Why then, as a general rule, has the impact of CPPs on medical practice been so limited thus far? First, physicians make clinical decisions by focusing on each individual patient they see, whereas CPPs focus instead on the entire population (i.e., the "average" patient). Physicians, therefore, may be skeptical of the data underlying particular CPPs (Gifford, 1996). In terms of outlining a flexible but carefully delineated range of acceptable practice for a particular problem, with constrained but adequate allowances for justified exceptions, a focus on broad populations rather than on every individual makes sense. By definition, most patients have to fall within an average range, and those whose medical needs deviate from that range are scarce rather than ordinary.

Second, many physicians want CPPs that are specific and concise enough that compliance will guarantee immunity against legal consequences for any bad patient result, but that at the same time allow the physician total discretion in patient care. Physicians must understand that this is an unreasonable expectation.

An important roadblock to physician compliance with CPPs is the prevalent mind-set, discussed earlier in several places, that "more is always better" in medicine. Although cost-containment initiatives surely can lead to the development and implementation of CPPs that have the effect of unduly jeopardizing patient health (Berger & Rosner, 1996; Morreim, 1995), physicians should resist the temptation to automatically dismiss certain ideas on the basis of disfavored sponsorship and motives rather than examining the content of those ideas.

Finally, much physician noncompliance with CPPs is the result of passive ignorance, as opposed to purposeful rejection. Resources invested in developing CPPs far outweigh those devoted to dissemination and education efforts. Many physicians welcome CPPs as support for themselves rather than seeing CPPs as a club aimed against them, but they often "forget" to utilize CPPs in everyday practice because their behavior is driven more by the availability of technology and associated financial incentives than by a true fear of liability.

Several factors are key to promoting physician practice that is consistent with relevant CPPs. First, physicians are more likely to embrace a CPP and thus more likely to comply with it if they have participated in some meaningful way in its development and adoption. This puts the onus on individual practitioners to participate in the process of creating policies, on the local and even particular institutional level, that reconcile or select among inconsistent or conflicting CPPs dealing with specific clinical subjects. The only way that physicians can break the vicious cycle of dependency on attorneys and the courts to resolve medical matters is to get seriously into the business of creating and implementing their own standards (Annas, 1994, p. 1545; Snider, 1995, p. 279).

Drafters of CPPs must use language that is clear, explicit, and comprehensible, yet precise enough to provide useful guidance for the physician. This is a challenging task, but one that is essential if the product is to be converted into behavior, with the consequent expected benefits in patient care, cost control, and legal risk management. Drafters also must make certain that the CPPs they develop are undeniably evidence-based and that this is apparent to potential users—especially physicians.

Finally, because passive ignorance is a major stumbling block to effective physician compliance with CPPs, one solution would be improved efforts at disseminating relevant CPPs and educating potential users about them. Although national dissemination initiatives are important, there is evidence that concentrated, focused education conducted at the local, organization-specific, peer-to-peer level are most effective in influencing tangible physician behavior. Medical and nursing staffs need to convey their endorsement of and commitment to their respective organizations' administration and governance regarding the development, adoption, and enforcement of appropriate CPPs. The organizational incentives for physicians must be consistent with the other forces attempting to influence their practice.

Informed Consent Implications

Some CPP proponents have suggested that consumers ought to be involved directly in the development of CPPs, or at least that CPPs should incorporate patient preferences (Oppenheim, Sotiropoulos, & Baraff, 1994). A much stronger argument can be made, however, for the physician's duty to inform individual patients (or their surrogates) about the existence and content of particular CPPs that are directly relevant to their own situations. In this manner, CPPs may be used to foster an atmosphere of better communication, partnership, and shared decision making about reasonable medical alternatives. Interestingly, when AHCPR itself was in the business of guideline development, it published two versions of each of its clinical practice guidelines—one written for health professionals and the other designed for lay consumers. Inevitably, the demand for consumer copies outstripped distribution of the professional version.

As discussed earlier, many physicians indicate that one of the most difficult tasks within the physician-patient relationship is explaining to the patient or surrogate why the physician is *not* ordering a particular diagnostic test or therapeutic intervention. For example, in a long-term-care facility a family might complain that the physician's failure to order physical or chemical restraints for a resident is unreasonably exposing that resident to an undue risk of injury. In such cases, the existence of professionally respected CPPs recommending only a very limited and judicious use of restraints may give the physician needed educational leverage with the family. In the final analysis, more informed consumer involvement almost always translates into better relationships, positive risk management, and a more favorable ethical environment within which to care for patients.

Changing the Medical Culture

Changing entrenched physician behavior will be very difficult and slow. There is a strong and persistent temptation for physicians to complain about the legal system's negative influence on medical ethics and to search for risk management survival "tricks" rather than to critically examine, with an eye toward improving, their own conduct. As one group of researchers into the causes of malpractice suits has noted, "What is troubling, however, is the possibility that some physicians may not recognize their weakness [in relating to patients] and simply see the current system of dispute resolution as unjust or at best random" (Hickson, Clayton, Entman, Miller, Githens, Whetten-Goldstein, & Sloan, 1994, p. 1587).

Influencing physician behavior in a more ethical direction will necessarily entail something fundamentally, qualitatively more than legislative tinkering, formal educational initiatives, and even CPP development and dissemination. Nothing less than a basic reexamination and reformation of the culture that permeates and shapes medical care will be necessary.

Although legal reforms may be desirable for numerous reasons, much ethical progress in medical conduct has occurred wholly independently of legal changes (Jayes, Zimmerman, Wagner, Draper, & Knaus, 1993) and many legal "improvements" have led to no discernible ethical progress. Similarly, although education is laudable in its own right, information alone does not necessarily create the belief environment of medicine that determines how physicians actually practice. As one author notes:

> The traditional pathway to behavior change has been seen as moving from changes in knowledge, to changes in attitude, and only then to changes in behavior. In fact, the reverse may be closer to the truth: change the environment and required (or socially approved) behaviors, and people's beliefs will adjust accordingly. (Solomon, 1995, p. S30)

Perceptions about liability exposure form one, but only one, significant facet of that whole, multidimensional change dynamic (Goldman, 1990).

The cultural expectations of medical practitioners must move away from the technology-worship, facts-for-their-own-sake, more-is-always-better aura that now characterizes most physicians' hearts and minds before meaningful behavioral modification will occur. The popular, even if unspoken, physician image of the patient's primary function as a source of scientific data for the clinician's decision making and/or intellectual curiosity must be dispelled, in favor of a relationship within which true power—and its accompanying responsibility—is shared. Physician egos also need to be readjusted over time, so that physicians no longer feel the need to criticize other practitioners in front of patients (e.g., "I'm glad you've come to me, because the guy you saw before really botched it"), and so that physicians will not be as fearful as many are today that their colleagues will level such criticisms against them directly to the patient.

The important influence of economic incentives on physician behavior cannot be ignored. Such incentives may be both real and symbolic. I have discerned a relatively relaxed attitude toward professional liability risk among salaried medical school faculty members, who feel that their employment status gives them a chance to devote sufficient time and interpersonal attention to their patients and/or their patients' families, as opposed to the more "uptight" atmosphere of full-time private practice. As noted many times earlier in this volume, money and organization not only talk loudly, but also in large ways drive physician behavior—negatively and positively—with a force often attributed, but usually wrongly, to legal liability anxieties. There is a strong consensus that physicians will treat patients in more ethically appropriate ways, regardless of the real state of the law, when unethical practice becomes more personally risky financially for the physician (Kapp, 1993a; Kapp, 1989b). Many versions of the sentiment, "Bad behavior needs to be deincentivised," have been declared as part of this discussion.

A RESEARCH AGENDA

As I have reported in these pages my own interpretation of the tensions between defensive medicine and good ethical patient care, I have shared my disappointment in several places that both individual physician practices and broad public policies too often proceed without adequate regard for—and sometimes in clear contradiction to—an accurate, relevant factual predicate. The quite limited research conducted to date on tort reform, for instance, has focused on legal system effects (e.g., impact on the size and outcome of malpractice lawsuits), while virtually ignoring the effects, if any, on the practice of defensive medicine and its implications for patient care (Bovbjerg, 1995). This situation needs to change, and the development and implementation of a substantial empirical research agenda could help greatly in the putting together of the sort of objective, evidence-based foundation upon which public policy relating to defensive medicine ought to be based.

Potential research questions measuring therapeutic jurisprudence—the tangible, positive impact of legal changes on human lives—abound. Is there, for example, some way that the statutory immunity against liability for physicians who volunteer to serve the poor—a strategy advocated by many as a matter of faith rather than data (Wurlitzer & McCool, 1994)—could be structured and presented so as to actually increase the number of physician volunteers? Does a physician's age have anything to do with how one handles anxiety about liability? For instance, do older physicians engage in less legally counterproductive and ethically questionable behavior than their younger counterparts? If so, is this because older physicians were not educated and socialized to believe in the magic and exclusivity of technology to the same extent as are today's cohort of medical students and residents; in other words, is it because older physicians were educated and socialized into the medical profession at a time when they had to spend time with and talk to patients because they had far less technology available? Or, as physicians acquire more experience, learning the limits and uncertainties of medicine and the importance of values in planning care, do they achieve a greater respect for the potential contribution that patients may be able to make by participating in their own health care decisions? Controlled demonstration projects and analyses of naturally occurring experiments could also provide policymakers and practitioners with clarifying data. For instance, more- and less-regulated health care environments could be compared on a variety of scales relating to the practice of defensive medicine and its impact on patient well-being.

The broad range of public and private interests with a significant stake in the ethical practice of medicine should be reflected in the governmental, foundation, and organizational entities willing to support such a research and demonstration agenda financially and through other forms of cooperation. This includes health and professional liability insurers, as well as institutional and organizational providers who are sincere about quality improvement in the ethical as well as other aspects of health care delivery.

CONCLUSION

For most physicians, how "courageous" they are on any particular day, in terms of not "caving in" to their liability anxieties, depends on how confident they feel that day and how tired they are at that moment of "running the legal and financial gauntlet" of modern medical practice. Others end up doing what they believe is "right" as much by default as by master plan, because they do not think anything they do will protect them from legal hassles anyway; if one is damned either way, they reason, physicians might just as well do the best they can and take their chances with the law (Taylor, 1994).

Physicians ought to act ethically in caring for their patients, but a medical ethics resulting from the physician having a "good day" or being reluctantly resigned to the vagaries of the liability lottery is morally weak and structurally unstable. I have tried in these pages to assist physicians, other health care providers, attorneys, and policy-makers to more knowledgeably appreciate—the better to constructively reconcile—the real and imagined tensions between fear of liability and defensive medicine, on one hand, and ethical medical practice on the other. It is my hope that a practice of medical ethics built on such a foundation and that addresses and resolves those tensions—a morally sincere and structurally enduring foundation—will inspire a medical ethics more worthy of the name for physicians, their patients, and society.

REFERENCES

Allery, L. A., Owen, P. A., & Robling, M. R. (1997). Why general practitioners and consultants change their clinical practice: A critical incident report. *British Medical Journal, 314*, 870–874.

American College of Physicians. (1995). Beyond MICRA: New ideas for liability reform. *Annals of Internal Medicine, 122*, 466–473.

American Medical Association. (1996). *Practice parameters: Titles, sources, and updates.* Chicago: AMA.

American Society of Health-System Pharmacists. (1995). Proceedings of a multidisciplinary invitational conference on understanding and preventing drug misadventures. *American Journal of Health-Systems Pharmacy, 52*, 369–417.

Annas, G. J. (1996). Facilitating choice: Judging the physician's role in abortion and suicide. *Quinnipiac Health Law Journal, 1*, 92–112.

Annas, G. J. (1995, November–December). How we lie. *Hastings Center Report, 25* (Special Supplement), S12–S14.

Annas, G. J. (1994). Asking the courts to set the standard of emergency care—the case of Baby K. *New England Journal of Medicine, 330*, 1542–1545.

Anonymous. (1996). Special report: Clinical practice guidelines. *Nursing Home Medicine, 1*.

Associated Press. (1996, July 1). Fla. malpractice suits down; tort reform gets credit. *American Medical News*, p. 8.

Bates, D. W., Leape, L. L., & Petrycki, S. (1993). Incidence and preventability of adverse events in hospitalized patients. *Journal of General Internal Medicine, 8*, 289–294.

Berger, J. T., and Rosner, F. (1996). The ethics of practice guidelines. *Archives of Internal Medicine, 156*, 2051–2056.

Berwick, D. M. (1989). Continuous improvement as an ideal in health care. *New England Journal of Medicine, 320*, 53–56.

Bogner, M. S. (1994). Human error in medicine: A frontier for change. In M.S. Bogner (Ed.), *Human Error in Medicine,* pp. 373–383. Hillsdale, NJ: Lawrence Erlbaum Associates.

Boohaker, E. A., Ward, R. E., Uman, J. E., & McCarthy, B. D. (1996). Patient notification and follow-up of abnormal test results. *Archives of Internal Medicine, 156,* 327–331.

Bosk, C. L. (1979). *Forgive and remember: Managing medical failure.* Chicago: University of Chicago Press.

Boumil, M. M., & Elias, C. E. (1995). *The law of medical liability.* St. Paul, MN: West Publishing Company.

Bovbjerg, R. (1995). *Medical malpractice: Problems and reforms — a policy-maker's guide to issues and information.* Washington, DC: Urban Institute Intergovernmental Health Project.

Bovbjerg, R. (1993). Medical malpractice: Research and reform. *Virginia Law Review, 79,* 2155–2208.

Brennan, T. A., & Berwick, D. M. (1996). *New Rules: Regulation, Markets, and the Quality of American Health Care.* San Francisco: Jossey-Bass Publishers.

Brown, L. C., & Procopio, J. (1995). Sailing through uncharted waters: Outcomes measurement, practice guidelines, and the law. *Whittier Law Review, 16,* 1021–1036.

Burn, S. (1996). Access to civil justice: Lord Woolf's visionary new landscape. *British Medical Journal, 313,* 242–243.

Butler, K. A. (1995). Health care quality revolution: Legal landmines for hospitals and the rise of the critical pathway. *Albany Law Review, 58,* 843–870.

Capron, A. M. (1995, May–June). Punishing medicine. *Hastings Center Report, 25,* 26–27.

Christensen, J. F., Levinson, W., and Dunn, P. M. (1992). The heart of darkness: The impact of perceived mistakes on physicians. *Journal of General Internal Medicine, 7,* 424–431.

Crowley, P. C. (1994). No pain, no gain? The Agency for Health Care Policy and Research's attempt to change inefficient health care practice of withholding medication from patients in pain. *Journal of Contemporary Health Law and Policy, 10,* 383–403.

Danzon, P. A. (1985). *Medical malpractice: Theory, evidence and public policy.* Cambridge, MA: Harvard University Press.

de Tocqueville, A. (1969). *Democracy in America.* G. Lawrence, trans.; J. P. Mayer, ed. New York: Doubleday Anchor.

Dillard, J. N. (1995, June 12). A doctor's dilemma: Helping an accident victim on the road could land you in court. *Newsweek,* p. 12.

Dyer, C. (1996). Overhaul of medical negligence litigation announced. *British Medical Journal, 313,* 247.

Ellrodt, A. G., Connor, L., Riedinger, M., & Weingarten, S. (1995). Measuring and improving physician compliance with clinical practice guidelines: A controlled interventional trial. *Annals of Internal Medicine, 122,* 277–282.

Ely, J. W. (1996). Physicians' mistakes: Will your colleagues offer support? *Archives of Family Medicine, 5,* 76–77.

Field, M. J. & Lohr, K. N. (Eds.). (1990). *Clinical practice guidelines: Directions for a new program.* Washington, DC: Institute of Medicine, National Academy Press.

Frisch, P. R., Charles, S. C., Gibbons, R. D., and Hedeker, D. (1995). Role of previous claims and specialty on the effectiveness of risk-management education for office-based physicians. *Western Journal of Medicine, 163,* 346–350.

Gifford, F. (1996, March/April). Outcomes research and practice guidelines: Upstream issues for downstream users. *Hastings Center Report, 26*(2), 38–44.

Goldman, L. (1990). Changing physicians' behavior: The pot and the kettle. *New England Journal of Medicine, 322,* 1524–1525.

Hall, M. A. (1991). The defensive effect of medical practice policies in malpractice litigation. *Law & Contemporary Problems, 54,* 119–145.

Hearn, W. (1996, April 1). Dueling guidelines: When is cholesterol screening needed? *American Medical News,* p. 13–14.

Hickson, G. B., Clayton, E. W., Entman, S. S., Miller, C. S., Githens, P. B., Whetten-Goldstein, K., & Sloan, F. A. (1994). Obstetricians' prior malpractice experience and patients' satisfaction with care. *Journal of the American Medical Association, 272,* 1583–1587.

Hilfiker, D. (1984). Facing our mistakes. *New England Journal of Medicine, 310,* 118–122.

Howard, S. K., Gaba, D. M., Fish, K. J., Yang, G., & Sarnquist, F. H. (1992). Anesthesia crisis resource management training: Teach anesthesiologists to handle critical incidents. *Aviation, Space & Environmental Medicine, 63,* 763–770.

Hubbard, F. P. (1989). The physicians' point of view concerning medical malpractice: A sociological perspective on the symbolic importance of "tort reform." *Georgia Law Review, 23,* 295–358.

Hyams, A. L., Brandenburg, J. A., Lipsitz, S. R., & Brennan, T. A. (1995). Practice guidelines and malpractice litigation: A two-way street. *Annals of Internal Medicine, 122,* 450–455.

Jayes, R. L., Zimmerman, J. E., Wagner, D. P., Draper, E. A., & Knaus, W. A. (1993). Do-not-resuscitate orders in intensive care units: Current practices and recent changes. *Journal of the American Medical Association, 270,* 2213–2217.

Johnson, H., & Broder, D. S. (1996). *The system: The American way of politics at the breaking point.* Boston: Little, Brown and Company.

Johnson, S. H. (1993, Fall). Law and quality in long-term care. *Journal of Long-Term Care Administration, 21,* 75–77.

Kadzielski, M., Weingarten, S., & Schroder, G. (1995). Peer review and practice guidelines under health care reform. *Whittier Law Review, 16,* 157–176.

Kapp, M. B. (1996). Therapeutic jurisprudence and end-of-life medical care: Physician perceptions of a statute's impact. *Medicine & Law, 15,* pp. 201–217.

Kapp, M. B. (1995). The legal status of clinical practice parameters: An updated annotated bibliography. *American Journal of Medical Quality, 10,* 107–111.

Kapp, M. B. (1993a, Spring). Informed consent to defensive medicine: Letting the patient decide. *Pharos of Alpha Omega Alpha, 56,* 12–14.

Kapp, M. B. (1993b). The legal status of clinical practice parameters: An annotated bibliography. *American Journal of Medical Quality, 8,* 24–27.

Kapp, M. B. (1990). The American medical malpractice system: Impediments to effective change. *International Journal of Risk and Safety in Medicine, 1,* 239–253.

Kapp, M. B. (1989a). Solving the medical malpractice problem: Difficulties in defining what works. *Law, Medicine & Health Care, 17,* 156–165.

Kapp, M. B. (1989b). Enforcing patient preferences: Linking payment for medical care to informed consent. *Journal of the American Medical Association, 261,* 1935–1938.

Katz, P. R., & Ouslander, J. G. (1996). Clinical practice guidelines and position statements: The American Geriatrics Society approach. *Journal of the American Geriatrics Society, 44,* 1123–1124.

Kessler, D., & McClellan, M. (1996). Do doctors practice defensive medicine? *Quarterly Journal of Economics, 111,* 353–390.

Kinney, E. (1995). Malpractice reform in the 1990s: Past disappointments, future success? *Journal of Health Politics, Policy and Law, 20,* 99–135.

Komaroff, A. L. (1987). Screening tests for nursing home patients. *Journal of the American Medical Association, 258,* 1941.

Lascaratos, J., & Dalla-Vorgia, P. (1996). Defensive medicine: Two historical cases. *International Journal of Risk and Safety in Medicine, 8,* 231–235.

Leape, L. L. (1994). Error in medicine. *Journal of the American Medical Association, 272,* 1851–1857.

Levinson, W. (1994). Physician-patient communication: A key to malpractice prevention. *Journal of the American Medical Association, 272,* 1619–1620.

Levinson, W., Roter, D. L., Mullooly, J. P., Dull, V. T., & Frankel, R. M. (1997). Physician-patient communication: The relationship with malpractice claims among primary care physicians and surgeons. *Journal of the American Medical Association, 277,* 553–559.

Levy, R. (1995, Fall). Code blue. *Harvard Public Health Review, 7,* 36–41.

McConkey, S. A., IV. (1995). Simplifying the law in medical malpractice: The use of practice guidelines as the standard of care in medical malpractice litigation. *West Virginia Law Review, 97,* 491–523.

McCrary, S. V., Swanson, J. W., Perkins, H. S., & Winslade, W. J. (1992). Treatment decisions for terminally ill patients: Physicians' legal defensiveness and knowledge of medical law. *Law, Medicine & Health Care, 20,* 364–376.

MMI Companies. (1996). *Monitoring quality, enhancing safety and managing healthcare risks in a time of change.* Deerfield, IL: MMI Companies.

Morreim, E. H. (1995). From advocacy to tenacity: Finding the limits. *Journal of the American Geriatrics Society, 43,* 1170–1172.

Morrissey, J. (1996, May 27). Risk management pays off-study. *Modern Healthcare, 26,* 34–36.

National Health Lawyers Association. (1995). *Colloquium report on legal issues related to clinical practice guidelines.* Washington, DC: NHLA.

North of England Asthma Guideline Development Group. (1996). North of England evidence based guidelines development project: Summary version of evidence based guidelines for the primary care management of asthma in adults. *British Medical Journal, 312,* 762–766.

Oppenheim, P. I., Sotiropoulos, G., & Baraff, L. J. (1994). Incorporating patient preferences into practice guidelines: Management of children with fever without source. *Annals of Emergency Medicine, 24,* 836–841.

Orentlicher, D. (1994a). The limits of legislation. *Maryland Law Review, 53,* 1255–1305.

Orentlicher, D. (1994b). The influence of a professional organization on physician behavior. *Albany Law Review, 57,* 583–605.

Perkins, H. S., Bauer, R. L., Hazuda, H. P., & Schoolfield, J. D. (1990). Impact of legal liability, family wishes, and other "external factors" on physicians' life-support decisions. *American Journal of Medicine, 89,* 185–194.

Petersen, S. K. (1995). No-fault and enterprise liability: The view from Utah. *Annals of Internal Medicine, 122,* 462–463.

Physician Insurers Association of America. (1996, May). *Acute myocardial infarction study.* Rockville, MD: PIAA.

Physician Payment Review Commission. (1994). *Annual report to Congress.* Washington, DC: PPRC.

Prager, L. O. (1996, November 4). Reducing medical errors. *American Medical News, 39* (1), 29.

Quill, T. E. (1994). Risk taking by physicians in legally gray areas. *Albany Law Review, 57,* 693–708.

Reid, M. C., Lachs, M. S., & Feinstein, A. R. (1995). Use of methodological standards in diagnostic test research: Getting better but still not good. *Journal of the American Medical Association, 274,* 645–651.

Richards, P., Kennedy, I. M., & Woolf, L. (1996). Managing medical mishaps: Needs greater openness and partnership between doctors, lawyers, judges, and patients. *British Medical Journal, 313,* 243–244.

Rinella, L. (1995). The use of medical practice guidelines in medical malpractice litigation—Should practice guidelines define the standard of care? *University of Missouri Kansas City Law Review, 64,* 337–355.

Rosoff, A. J. (1995). The role of clinical practice guidelines in health care reform. *Health Matrix, 5,* 369–396.

Saks, M. (1992). Do we really know anything about the behavior of the tort litigation system—and why not? *University of Pennsylvania Law Review, 140,* 1147–1292.

Sarwar, A. (1996). Guidelines in need of guidance. *Chest, 109,* 594–595.

Schmitt, R. B. (1995, March 7). Truth is first casualty of tort-reform debate. *Wall Street Journal,* p. B1.

Schriger, D. L. (1996). Emergency medicine clinical guidelines: We can make them, but will we use them? *Annals of Emergency Medicine, 27,* 655–657.

Schwartz, J. S., & Shulkin, D. J. (1995). Teaching an old dog new tricks. *Journal of General Internal Medicine, 10,* 353–354.

Seal of approval [Editorial]. (1996). *American Medical News,* p. 17.

Shuman, D. W. (1993). The psychology of deterrence in tort law. *Kansas Law Review, 42,* 115–168.

Snider, G. L. (1995). Withholding and withdrawing life-sustaining therapy: All systems are not yet "go." *American Journal of Respiratory and Critical Care Medicine, 151,* 279–281.

Solomon, M. Z. (1995, November–December). The enormity of the task: SUP-
PORT and changing practice. *Hastings Center Report, 25* (Suppl.), S28–S32.

Taler, G. (1996). Clinical practice guidelines: Their purposes and uses. *Journal of
the American Geriatrics Society, 44,* 1108–1111.

Taylor, W. G. (1994). A patient's choice? [Letter]. *Western Journal of Medicine, 161,*
526–527.

U.S. Congress, Office of Technology Assessment. (1994). *Defensive medicine and
medical malpractice.* Washington, DC: U.S. Government Printing Office.

U.S. Department of Health and Human Services. (1987, August). *Report of the task
force on medical liability and malpractice.* Washington, DC: DHHS.

Webster, J. R., Jr. (1995). Geriatrics practice guidelines not a cookbook. *Center on
Aging* (Buehler Center on Aging, McGaw Medical Center, Northwestern
University), *11*(3), 1–2.

Weiler, P. C. (1995). Fixing the tail: The place of malpractice in health care reform.
Rutgers Law Review, 47, 1157–1193.

Weiler, P. C. (1991). *Medical malpractice on trial.* Cambridge, MA: Harvard University Press.

Wertz, D. C., Fanos, J. H., & Reilly, P. R. (1994). Genetic testing for children and
adolescents: Who decides? *Journal of the American Medical Association, 272,*
875–881.

Williams, P. C., & Winslade, W. J. (1995). Educating medical students about law
and the legal system. *Academic Medicine, 70,* 777–786.

Wurlitzer, F., & McCool, R. (1994). Legal immunity for physician volunteers
[Letter]. *Journal of the American Medical Association, 272,* 31.

Index

Access to health care, 28–29, 41–43, 125
Administrative officials, health care, 4
Adult protective services, 111
Advance medical directives, 61, 76–77, 145
Advertising, 4
Age, physician's as factor in behavior, 163
Agency for Healthcare Policy and Research (AHCPR), 154, 160
Alternative Dispute Resolution (ADR), 143
Alzheimer's disease patients, driving by, 117
American Academy of Hospital Attorneys (AAHA), 54
American Association for the Advancement of Science (AAAS), 148
American College of Physicians, 33
American Geriatrics Society, 87
American Heart Association, 68–69, 87n.1
American Medical Association, 32, 74, 79, 135, 148, 154
American Medical Directors Association, 154

American Society for Healthcare Risk Management (ASHRM), 54
Americans With Disabilities Act (ADA), 84
Annenberg Center for Health Sciences, 148
Antitrust, 131, 135
Art of medicine, 35
Assisted living, 103–04
Autonomy, patient, 28, 65, 104–07, 110, 112, 114; informed consent implications, 36–40; restraints, 99, 100, 102
Autonomy, physician, 131–32, 135
Autopsies, 41

Baby Doe controversy, 61, 68
Barber case, 78–79
Beneficence, 28, 40, 57, 99, 100, 106, 110, 112
Blue Cross/Blue Shield, 126
Bohlmann case, 85
Breast cancer, 38

Capacity assessments, 108–110
Cardiopulmonary resuscitation (CPR), 68–
   70, 75–76
Care standards, 7, 20
Case management, 111
"Catastrophobia," 98
Certification, 85, 131
Cesarean sections, 30, 33
Child abuse and neglect, 68
Cholesterol screening, 157
Clinical Laboratory Improvement Amend-
   ments (CLIA), 43, 131
Clinical practice parameters, 113, 153–160
Clinton health care reform plan, 127, 156
Coalition for Quality End-of-Life Care, 74
"Code of Silence," 148
Collegiality, medical, 35, 130, 162
Commitment, involuntary, 116–117
Communications, 36–40, 75, 152
Community health centers, 42
Competency. See Capacity assessments.
Competitive medical marketplace, 3, 4, 5,
   39, 135
Consent: forms, 38; informed, 34, 36–40,
   108–10, 160
Conservatorship. See Guardianship.
Consumers Union, 131
Controlled substances. See Pain treatment
Consultants, specialty, 36
Coronary procedures, 36
Criminal prosecution, fear of, 78–81
Critically ill patients. See Dying patients,
   treatment of
Cruzan case, 81

Dangerous patients, 116–117
Data: consumer access to, 123, 131–132; ef-
   fect of risk management, 153; malprac-
   tice system, 11, 144–45, 162–63
"Defensive law," 57
Defensive medicine, definition and mea-
   surement, 28, 29–34
Devices, access to, 43
Diagnosis Related Groups (DRGs), 128, 157
Diagnostic tests. See Overtesting
Discrimination in treatment. See Ameri-
   cans With Disabilities Act
Documentation, 35–36, 37, 153

Do-not-resuscitate (DNR) orders. See Car-
   diopulmonary resuscitation
Drake Center, 97–98
Drugs, access to, 43, 135
Durable powers of attorney, 115. See also
   Advance medical directives
Dying patients, treatment of, 17, 58, 65–
   87, 145

Education, medical. See Medical educa-
   tion.
Einaugler case, 79–80
Electronic fetal monitoring, 30
Emergency medical system (EMS), 70
Emotional costs of being sued, 9–10, 144
End-of-life care. See Dying patients, treat-
   ment of
Enterprise liability, 143
"Episodic panic," 98
Errors, medical, 2, 20–22, 40–41, 147–49
Ethics committees, 61–63
Etiology, physician anxieties, 2, 12–20
Euthanasia. See Dying patients, treatment
   of
Expenditures, health care, 28, 42, 124–27,
   134, 154–55

Family: consent statutes, 76; as potential
   plaintiffs, 82–83, 108; physicians, 30
Federal Aviation Administration (FAA)
   model, 147
Federal Tort Claims Act, 42
Federally Supported Health Centers As-
   sistance Act, 42
Feeding and hydration, artificial, 70–72,
   76, 80, 85–86
Fidelity, 41
Financial costs of being sued, 8, 144
Financial incentives, 75, 110, 127, 130, 132–
   37, 143, 146, 162. See also Competitive
   medical marketplace
Financial institutions, 115
Financing, health care, 124–132
Food and Drug Administration (FDA),
   99–100, 101–02
Fraud and abuse, 32, 46n.1, 131
Freedom of Information Act (FOIA), 102
Futile treatment, 68, 84, 85, 87

Gallant case, 85
Good Samaritan statutes, 43, 146
Government *qua* health insurance purchaser, 125–26
Guardianship, 107–16; alternatives to, 110–16

"Hanging crepe," 38
Health maintenance organizations (HMOs), 129
Health Security Act of 1994. *See* Clinton health care reform plan
Home- and community-based long term care, 104–107
Hospitals, restraints in, 100–102
Hydration, artificial. *See* Feeding and hydration, artificial

Immunity, legal, 66, 146–47
Indigent. *See* Poor people
Innovation, medical, 43–44
Insurance: health, 123, 125–30, 163; liability, 8, 10, 20, 27–28, 29, 110–12, 115, 147, 163
Internal Revenue Code, 126
International comparisons, 33, 43, 124, 150, 153
Interpersonal relationships, 31, 75

Joint Commission on Accreditation of Healthcare Organizations (JCAHO), 61, 69, 102, 131, 148
Justice, social or distributive, 28–29, 42

Kramp case, 77, 82

Laboratories, clinical, 43, 131
Landers, Ann, 80
"Last Acts" project, 75
Lawsuits, physicians' fear of, 8–10, 112, 113–14
"Learned helplessness," 104, 106
Least restrictive alternative principle, 109
Legal counsel, in-house, 12, 53–64, 77, 82, 112–13, 152
"Legal denial," 55
"Legisogenic" treatment, 67
Licensure, 85, 131, 149

Life support, discontinuation of, 17, 58, 70–87, 145
Literature, medicolegal, 14–17, 151
Living wills. *See* Advance medical directives

Malaise, psychological, of physicians, 123–137
"Malpractice stress syndrome," 10
Managed care, 4, 33, 128–30, 132, 133–37
Managed risk. *See* Negotiated risk
Massachusetts, legislation on consumer access to data, 123, 131
Maternity care, 30, 40, 42–43
Medicaid, 32, 85, 124–25, 127–28, 131, 136
Medical culture, changing, 161–162
Medical education: continuing, 19, 150–52; mandatory risk management component, 56, 153; postgraduate, 18–19, 43, 151; undergraduate, 14, 17–18, 43, 124, 151
"Medical grapevine," 12–14
Medical records. *See* Documentation
Medical Society of the State of New York, 79
Medicare, 32, 85, 124–25, 127–28, 131, 136, 157
Mental health, 116–17
Messenger case, 68
Money management services, 111, 115
"Moral tutor," role of law as, 45
Mortality and morbidity (M&M) conferences, 40
"My last case" syndrome, 158

National Patient Safety Foundation, 148–149
National Practitioner Data Bank (NPDB), 9–10, 131
Natural death legislation, 76–77, 145
Negative test results, 37
Neglect and abuse, 104, 105, 114
Negotiated risk, 104
Newborns. *See* Baby Doe controversy
New York, DNR statute, 75–76
No-fault system, 143
Nonmaleficence, 28, 40, 57, 99, 100, 110, 141
Nursing homes, 71, 85, 86, 99–100, 109–10; Nursing Home Quality Reform Act, 99, 101

Nutrition. *See* Feeding and hydration, arti-
    ficial

Obstetrics. *See* Maternity care
Oncologists, 5–6
Ophthalmology, 39–40
Organ donation. *See* Transplantation
Overtesting, 34–36
Overtreatment, 36

Pain treatment, 72–75, 81, 87
Palliative care. *See* Pain treatment
Paramedics, 70
Paternalistic behavior, 98, 103, 105–06
Patient expectations, physicians' percep-
    tions of, 3, 5, 39, 133
Patient Self-Determination Act (PSDA),
    61, 69
Payouts, malpractice, 11
Pediatrics, 42
Physical costs of being sued, 10
Physician/patient relationship, 41, 130,
    134, 152–53
Poor people, 42–43, 146–47, 163
Practice guidelines. *See* Clinical practice
    parameters
Preferred provider organizations (PPOs),
    129
Preoperative workup, 35
Pretext, law as, 4, 30–32, 34, 115, 135–37,
    145, 150; capacity assessments, 108–
    109; end-of-life context, 83–84; re-
    straints,   102
Primum non nocere. *See* Nonmaleficence
Prospective payment, 127–128
Prostate specific antigen (PSA), 39
Proxies. *See* Surrogate decision makers
Psychiatrists, 42, 116–17
Public Citizen Health Research Group,
    131
Public Health Service, 42
Publicity, fears of, 8, 112, 114, 132

Quality assurance mechanisms, 131–32,
    149, 154
Quinlan case, 81

Radio, 14–15

Rationalization. *See* Pretext, law as
Reading, by physicians, 14–17, 151
Regulatory sanctions, fear of, 84–85
Representative payees, 111, 115
Research agenda, 162–163
Research, biomedical, 43
"Resident mentality," 31, 33
Restraints, 70, 98–102, 160
Retirement, physicians' early, 135
Right to die issues. *See* Dying patients,
    treatment of
Right to die litigation rate, 86–87
Risk management: education, 152–153;
    products, 20
Risk managers, 12, 53–64, 77, 152
Robert Wood Johnson Foundation, 65, 75
Rural areas, 43

Safe Medical Devices Act (SMDA), 100,
    102
Social Security Administration, 115
Standards, 113. *See also* Care standards.
Stress. *See* Emotional costs of being sued
Suicide, physician-assisted, 73–74, 87
Support Services for Elders, 111
SUPPORT study, 65–66
Surgery, 39–40
Surrogate decision makers, 109
"Swing beds," 101

Tabloids, 14–16, 132
Tax Equity and Fiscal Responsibility Act
    (TEFRA), 128
Technological imperative, 32, 33, 161–162
Television, 14–15
Test results, abnormal, 152
"Theory of Bad Apples," 155
Therapeutic jurisprudence, 162–163
Tort system, attitudes toward, 6–8, 11, 44,
    142–43, 161; compensation function, 45;
    deterrence value of, 7, 41–42, 44–45; re-
    form, 142–50
Transfers, patient, 85
Transplantation, 57–58, 83

Uncertainty, medical, 2, 22, 31, 34–35

Vaccinations, 42

Veterans Affairs, Department of, 115, 124
Violent and suicidal patients, 42
Volunteer programs, 43, 115, 163
VQ scan, 35

Wall Street Journal, 79–80, 144

Wasteful medicine, 28, 42, 136
Welby, Marcus, 127
Wickline case, 133–134
Wilson case, 134

X rays, 35

ABOUT THE AUTHOR

MARSHALL B. KAPP has degrees in Public Health and in Law. He is a professor in the departments of Community Health and Psychiatry and Director, Office of Geriatric Medicine and Gerontology, Wright State University School of Medicine. He is a member of the adjunct faculty at the University of Dayton School of Law. He serves as editor of the *Journal of Ethics, Law, and Aging* and has written numerous books, including *Geriatrics and the Law* (second edition, 1992) and *Preventing Malpractice in Long Term Care* (1987).